Understanding Aging and Diversity

The demographic phenomena of increased life expectancy, increasing global population of older adults, and a larger number of older people as a proportion of the total population in nations throughout the world will affect our lives and the life of each person we know. The changes will result in challenges and benefits for societies and people of all ages. These events need to be understood, explained, and their consequences addressed; sociological theories about aging are an essential part of this process.

In *Understanding Aging and Diversity: Theories and concepts*, Patricia Kolb presents important sociological theories and concepts for understanding experiences of older people and their families in a rapidly changing world. She explores concepts from phenomenology, critical theory, feminist theory, life course theory and gerotranscendence theory to explain important issues in the lives of older people. This book investigates similarities and differences in aging experiences, focusing in particular on the effects of inequality. Kolb examines the relationship of ethnicity, race, gender, sexual orientation and social class to international aging experiences.

This book explores the relationships between older people and social systems in different ways, and informs thinking about policy development and other strategies for enhancing the wellbeing of older adults. It will be useful for students and scholars of sociology, gerontology, social work, anthropology, economics, demography, global studies, and political science.

Patricia Kolb is Associate Professor in the Department of Social Work at Lehman College, City University of New York.

Routledge advances in sociology

Understanding Aging and Diversity

Theories and concepts

Patricia Kolb

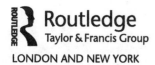

Routledge
Taylor & Francis Group

LONDON AND NEW YORK

First published 2014 by Routledge

2 Park Square, Milton Park, Abingdon, Oxfordshire OX14 4RN
52 Vanderbilt Avenue, New York, NY 10017

Routledge is an imprint of the Taylor & Francis Group, an informa business

First issued in paperback 2019

British Library Cataloguing in Publication Data
A catalogue record for this book is available from the British Library

Library of Congress Cataloging-in-Publication Data
Kolb, Patricia J.
   Understanding aging and diversity : theories and concepts / Patricia Kolb.
   pages cm. — (Routledge advances in sociology; 113)
   Includes bibliographical references and index.
   1. Gerontology. 2. Older people—Social conditions. 3. Aging. 4. Aging—
Cross-cultural studies. I. Title
HQ1061.K643 2013
305.26—dc23

                                                              2013007128

ISBN: 978-0-415-67881-0 (hbk)
ISBN: 978-0-367-86628-0 (pbk)

Typeset in TimesNewRomanPSMT
by Cenveo Publisher Services

This book is dedicated to my sisters, Teresa L. Altemeyer and Jeannette Kniesly Kralovansky, with respect and appreciation for their caring friendships with older people.

Contents

Figures

Acknowledgments

I am extremely fortunate to have received support in my work on this book from many people. I am grateful that when I contacted Routledge with the idea of writing a book about theoretical perspectives for understanding aging and diversity for their Advances in Sociology series, the response from sociology publisher Gerhard Boomgaarden was extremely positive. I appreciate his understanding of the importance of this book and support throughout this process, as well as the assistance of editorial assistants Emily Briggs and Jennifer Dodd. I am also grateful for recommendations from the proposal and manuscript reviewers.

I appreciate opportunities that I have been given in the past by John Michel, Sonia Austrian, Colleen Galambos, and Sherry Cummings to write about gerontological theories and diversity. I am also grateful for the superb educational background in sociological theory that I received as a student at the New School for Social Research, particularly from Dr. Stanford M. Lyman.

I am grateful for the exceptional support for writing this book that I have received from Dr. Norma Phillips, Chair of the Department of Social Work at Lehman College, City University of New York. I am also very appreciative for the opportunities provided by Dr. Madeline Moran, former Chairperson of the Sociology Department at Lehman College, to develop and teach an undergraduate course about sociological theories of aging, and Dr. Elin Waring, current Chairperson of the Sociology Department for providing the opportunity for me to teach the course again in 2012. The support of my colleagues in the Department of Social Work for my work on this book and my sabbatical fellowship leave during the fall, 2011, semester has been invaluable for completion of this book in a timely manner. I am grateful to the administration of Lehman College for granting my request for the leave.

The students who I have taught in the Sociological Theories of Aging course have provided very important feedback that has been incorporated into my work on this book. My meetings about gerotranscendence with Lars Tornstam and Jannie Pevik Fasth in Uppsala, and opportunities to learn from Timothy Stayton and his colleagues and members of the older adults group in Eskilstuna provided valuable learning opportunities during my research trip to Sweden. The interest and confidence that Karen and Fred Muir, Bernice Berk, and Alexis Hill have shown for my writing has been very important, and I appreciate the patience and confidence of my son, Anthony, during my work on this book.

1 Introduction

Key Concepts

1. The demographic phenomena of increased life expectancy, increasing global population of older adults, and a larger number of older people as a proportion of the total population in nations throughout the world will result in challenges and benefits for societies and people of all ages.
2. Demographic realities require that we educate ourselves and others about demographic changes; understand and analyze their implications for individuals, social institutions, and entire societies; and address related needs of individuals and social systems.
3. Sociological theories aid our understanding of aging experiences of diverse older adults and their families, communities, and societies as they experience social changes resulting from current demographic realities and develop plans for the future.
4. Theorizing involves developing ideas that assist in prediction and understanding and explaining empirical observations.
5. Knowledge about demographic transition, a process that occurs when increased life expectancy and declining fertility rates drive population aging, helps us to understand why the proportion of older adults in nations throughout the world is increasing.
6. Biological, psychological, spiritual, and social changes occur as people age in different environments, and variations exist in the experiences of individuals and groups throughout life.
7. Cohort differences, such as changes in women's roles, contribute to diversity of experiences of older adults and introduce new challenges and benefits for families and communities.
8. Experiences related to inequality, oppression, and privilege occur within cultural contexts and are powerful determinants of quality of life in later adulthood.
9. Active aging is defined by the World Health Organization (WHO) as "the process of optimizing opportunities for health, participation, and security in order to enhance quality of life as people age" (WHO 2002: 2).

Introduction

Chapter 1 provides a foundation for discussion of theoretical perspectives and theories in this book by providing an introduction to historical and sociological perspectives on aging, demographic changes, social effects of these changes, and the concept of diversity in aging experiences. The World Health Organization (WHO) concept of "active aging" and its determinants are presented.

The importance of sociological theories of aging

> There is precedent neither for the ageing of the world's population nor for the solutions to the problems such a demographic upheaval creates. The task cuts across generations, international borders, and the boundaries of traditional economic and political institutions. It calls for new ways of thinking, an enlarged sense of social responsibility, and a willingness to imagine and create something for which there is no blueprint.
>
> (Alvarez 1999: 2)

Demographic realities require that we educate ourselves and others about the changes; understand and analyze their implications for individuals, social institutions, and entire societies; and address related needs of individuals and social systems. Sociological theories aid our understanding of aging experiences of diverse older adults and their families, communities, and societies as they experience social changes resulting from contemporary demographic realities and develop plans for the future. The demographic phenomena of increased life expectancy, increasing global population of older adults, and a larger number of older people as a proportion of the total population in nations throughout the world will affect our lives and the life of each person we know. The changes will result in challenges and benefits for societies and people of all ages. These events need to be understood, explained, and their consequences addressed, and sociological theories about aging are an essential part of this process.

How can sociological theory help us to understand and respond to the "agequake" and its consequences? In reality, theorizing about aging is familiar to us because we are accustomed to developing our own theories to explain everyday observations about aging. As we interact with older people, we theorize about observed changes and consistencies in individuals and groups. We consider older people within the context of social institutions and structures. How have social circumstances affected the older person's life? What is the person's socioeconomic status and how did this develop? How did the older person's support systems develop? What are the limits to the support that can be provided by family and community? What is the appropriate role of government in responding to the needs of older people?

We theorize about whether older people and their relatives' current situations have been affected by institutional discrimination or a history of unearned or earned privilege and theorize about their future. Do people in the person's potential support system appear to be disproportionately affected by illness and therefore limited in their capacity to provide assistance? Is good health pervasive in the support system? We might theorize that the person is simply lucky or unlucky, or influenced by "good" or "bad" genes, or think sociologically about whether institutional influences have played an important role in the older person's life circumstances. Our theories about causation will affect our theorizing about solutions to problems that we perceive, including institutional impediments to achieving optimum functioning in later adulthood.

Theory has been defined as "the construction of explicit explanations that account for empirical findings." Stated another way, "answers to...'why' and 'how' questions require theory, which is *an attempt to explain.*" Theorizing is "a process of *developing ideas that allow us to understand and explain empirical observations.*" Features of theory that remain constant are theory as an attempt to explain, theorizing as a process, and the requirement that theorizing be explicit, not implicit or covert (Bengtson et al. 2009: 3–5). Theoretical perspectives provide orientations for developing theories.

This book exists because of the author's belief that sociological theories of aging are essential contributions to the knowledge base for understanding and responding to social changes related to demography and diversity in aging experiences. The global community needs answers to many age-related questions, and theorists have developed ideas to explain observations about aging. What ideas exist about approaches for responding to global changes related to aging? What can we anticipate from individuals, families and other social institutions, and communities on various levels within the contexts of different histories, social structures, cultures, values, traditions, and technological resources? How can we prepare for a future with the challenges of a global "agequake?"

The changing world: demographic projections

You and I experience aging on an individual and social basis daily in multiple ways that directly affect our lives and the experiences of everyone that we know. At the highest end of the age continuum, you may know people who are in their eighties, nineties, or centenarians who have lived more than one hundred years. According to the World Health Organization, from 2006 to 2050 the proportion of people age 60 and over will increase from 11 percent to 22 percent of the global population. This will result in the unprecedented phenomenon of a larger worldwide older adult population than number of children up to the age of 14 (WHO 2007).

Increases in older people as a percentage of the total population within nations are anticipated in all countries except in sub-Saharan Africa (Kalache et al. 2005). Significant regional differences are projected. Twenty-one percent of the population in more developed regions is aged 60 and over, and it is projected that in 2050 that proportion of the population will be 33 percent. In developing countries as a whole, 8 percent of the population is age 60 and over, but by 2050 that proportion will be 20 percent (UN 2009: viii).

In the United States, the population of people age 65 and over increased by 15.1 percent from 2000 to 2010 compared to a total population increase of 9.7 percent. There continues to be a greater proportion of older females compared to older males, but a pronounced increase in the number of older males diminished the gap during this decade (Werner 2011). It is projected that there will be twice as many people age 65 and over in 2030 as there were in 2008, resulting in a population of about 72.1 million older adults in 2030 (Greenberg 2009).

There are projected subgroup variations in the increase in the percentage of older people within countries. In the United States, the percentage of older adults belonging to racial and ethnic minority groups will increase faster than the percentage of Caucasian older adults. In 2030, minority populations are projected to be 25.4 percent of the population 65 years and older, an increase from 17.2 percent in 2002. From 2000 to 2030, the White population age 65 and older is projected to increase by 77 percent while the older Hispanic population is projected to increase by 342 percent, the older African American proportion of the population is projected to increase by 164 percent, the older American Indian, Eskimo, and Aleutian population by 207 percent, and Asian and Pacific Islander older population by 302 percent (Dilworth-Anderson and Cohen 2009).

Knowledge about demographic transition helps us to understand why the proportion of older adults in nations throughout the world is increasing. This is a process that occurs when increased life expectancy and declining fertility rates drive population aging. This process is progressing much more rapidly in developing countries than it has historically in nations that are now more highly developed. The differences in the length of time for the population age 65 and over to increase from 7 percent to 14 percent of a nation's population have been dramatic. For example, it took 115 years, from 1865 to 1980, for the proportion of the population that was age 65 and over to double in France. Doubling took 85 years, from 1890 to 1972, in Sweden. In contrast, the proportion of the population age 65 and older in South Korea is expected to double in 18 years, from 2000 to 2018. Similarly, it is projected that in Singapore doubling will take 19 years, from 2000 to 2019, and 19 years in Colombia, from 2017 to 2036 (Kinsella and He 2009: 14). In the U.S., the population age 65 and over increased from 3.1 million in 1900 to 40.3 million in 2010 (Werner 2011).

The fastest growing age group in most, if not all, highly industrialized countries includes people who are age 85 and older, described as the "oldest-old" (Poon et al. 2005). They are about 1 percent of the global population and 17 percent of the older adult population, constituting 22 percent of the older population in developed countries and 13 percent in less developed countries (Poon et al. 2005: 346). Over half of the people who are in this age group live in China, Germany, India, Japan, the Russian Federation, and the U.S. (Poon et al. 2005: 346). In the United States, the majority of the oldest old population is in the 85 to 89 year old age group, but the largest percentage point increase between 1990 and 2010 among people age 85 and over was in the 90 to 94 year old age group (Werner 2011).

Sociodemographic characteristics that differentiate the oldest-old from the young-old include greater likelihood of living alone, especially for females;

increased likelihood of institutionalization; lower levels of education and higher poverty rates; and the likelihood of increased racial and ethnic diversity. Nevertheless, people 85 and older vary widely in their health and functioning, with approximately one-third living independently, one-third functionally impaired, and one-third extremely disabled (Poon et al. 2005: 346–7).

Societal effects of demographic changes

Evidence presented at the United Nations Second World Assembly on Ageing in Madrid in 2002 predicted that the effects of unprecedented demographic changes will be experienced in:

> economic growth, savings, investment and consumption, labour markets, pensions, taxation and the transfers of wealth, property and care from one generation to another. Population aging will continue to affect health and health care, family composition and living arrangements, housing and migration. In the political arena, population aging has already produced a powerful voice in developed countries, as it can influence voting patterns and representation. Older voters usually read, watch the news, educate themselves about the issues, and they vote in much higher percentages than any other age group.
>
> (UN 2002b: 1)

Socioeconomic consequences include the need for alterations in public and private pension plans due to changes in age and employment structures (Kalache et al. 2005). Simultaneously, population aging and the increasing participation of women in the paid labor force are factors diminishing the capacity of family members to be caregivers for older relatives (Kalache et al. 2005; Kolb 2003). Severe shortages of trained health care workers to provide services to older adults will continue in both developed and developing nations (Kalache et al. 2005; Kolb 2003; Stone and Wiener 2001). Additional issues that need to be addressed include health and health care, income support, elder abuse, employment for older adults, HIV/AIDS in older people, employment and voluntary action by older people, and safety for older migrants and refugees (UN 2002b).

Health care policy makers will need to address results of epidemiological transition, the transition from predominance of disease and death resulting from infectious diseases to increased prevalence of disease and death resulting from non-communicable diseases. This transition is occurring much more rapidly in developing nations than the historically slower durations in developed nations. This shift is a societal achievement, but will present challenges for developing countries in which infectious diseases such as malaria and tuberculosis, and more recently identified diseases such as HIV and AIDS, will continue to exist at high levels concurrently with increased prevalence of non-communicable diseases. For example, in Botswana in sub-Saharan Africa, life expectancy is declining because of premature death of children and young adults, while the older adult proportion of the population has increased or remained stable because the older population's risk for HIV is lower. Health care systems in developing countries will be challenged to meet the needs of an increasing population of older adults in addition to addressing health care needs of younger people (Kalache et al. 2005).

Although there are challenges, benefits will also result from population aging. In Asia and Latin America, current demographic pressures on land are expected to diminish with the decline in the number of young people and stabilization in the number of adults (UN 2002a: 3). Older people are sources of skill, experience, and support to family members, friends, and their communities. Globally, approximately 16 million children age 15 and younger have lost one or both parents to AIDS; 29 countries in sub-Saharan Africa, three in Asia, and two in Latin America and the Caribbean have been most severely affected by HIV and AIDS (Kalache et al. 2005: 39). Slightly older brothers and sisters and grandparents are the primary caregivers for these children, and in Zambia, Uganda, and Tanzania the largest group of caregivers for orphans is grandparents (Kalache et al. 2005). While this caregiving is invaluable, resources are needed to support older people who are caregivers. In the U.S., millions of older people, especially older women, provide care informally in their communities in addition to over three million older people who work as volunteers in health and political organizations, schools, and religious organizations (Kalache et al. 2005).

In discussing the strengths of older adults, it is important to acknowledge that the oldest-old, people 85 and over, have unique strengths. Poon et al. (2005: 349, 352), write that:

> Since ageing itself is an adaptational process, the oldest-old have advantages in dealing with stresses and developing efficient personal coping strategies through lifetime experiences. It is also suggested that the oldest-old have differential expectations and perspectives of life and lowered reference points based on realities in advanced old age (C.L. Johnson and Barer, 1997). An example would be that the oldest-old are more likely to consider disease and disability as changes with ageing rather than health problems. Finally, the oldest-old may benefit from selective survivorship. Their special status as survivors beyond the expected lifespan may bolster psychological states of the oldest-old and help them make positive evaluations of themselves (Martin et al., 2000; Poon et al., 1992b)....The profiles of the oldest-old show both continuity and discontinuity. Perhaps the diversities and paradoxes of living to be the oldest-old demonstrate a resiliency of the human spirit, and much of that resiliency remains to be understood.

Diversity in aging experiences

Cohort and cultural differences and similarities

In this book, theories and research studies are discussed with regard to their implications for understanding diversity of experiences in aging. Biological, psychological, spiritual, and social changes occur as people age in different environments, and variations exist in the experiences of individuals and groups throughout life. These include cohort and cultural differences. While some influential events occur locally, others are global phenomena, including the contemporary "agequake," economic downturns, and decrease and increase in prevalence of diseases such as HIV/AIDS that affect people of all ages.

Cohort differences, such as changes in women's roles, contribute to diversity of experiences of older adults and introduce new challenges and benefits for families and communities. In some countries, these changes have provided new employment and income opportunities for women that result in more substantial financial resources in later adulthood. However, changes in women's employment, income, and marital options such as divorce can reduce time available for women, often the traditional caregivers for older relatives and neighbors, to assist older people in need.

In some families in Kolb's (2003) study of nursing home residents and their relatives and friends in a large city in the U.S., cohort changes in roles available to women reduced availability of females to be caregivers for older relatives. When women and men in the family and friendship groups could not provide adequate informal assistance and publicly funded and privately paid assistance was inadequate to meet the needs, nursing home placement resulted. Kolb (2003: 15) notes that:

> ...demographic data clearly indicate that structural changes are affecting families on a large scale in the United States. With increasing longevity, a larger number of individuals eventually need assistance from informal or formal service providers, or both. The changes noted – more older people needing assistance, more women in the labor force, and more divorces – make it difficult for families to provide sufficient care. As the daughter of [a]...nursing home resident...said, 'I know that she requires a lot of care, and we all work and I don't think we'd be able to take care of her.'

Cultural contexts also influence responses to shared events. Dilworth-Anderson and Cohen (2009) propose that the challenging task of theorizing across cultures in later life is facilitated by using a culturally competent theorizing process or approach. They consider cultural metaphors and values to be fundamentals for a culturally competent process and believe that metaphors help us to understand behavior and interaction of cultural groups. In their discussion of metaphors, they write that:

> Different cultural groups use distinct metaphors to express their experiences which often have historical connections that are passed from one generation to the next within a culture. In the African American culture, for example, the circle has represented both the confinement of bondage and a sense of belonging within their cultural community.... The fence, another

metaphor of some cultural groups, sets limits about who comes in and who is kept out.

(Dilworth-Anderson and Cohen 2009: 488)

Dilworth-Anderson and Cohen (2009: 488) believe that "cultural values of a group can give more concrete meaning to the metaphors when theorizing across cultures in later life." They write:

> Cultural values can inform theorizing across cultural groups because they provide an understanding of 'being' for a people....[Values] are standards that guide individual actions, even though they may change over time because of individual, group, historical, and societal factors. They give us more than insight; they provide some explanation and understanding of a persons [sic] or group's life. Values also provide direction for behavior and give parameters for acceptable and unacceptable behavior within groups. They also tell us what to expect of ourselves and what to expect of others within our primary groups, such as families. Similar to metaphors, values provide an understanding of how individuals experience themselves and others....Thus, metaphors provide images and meanings, and values provide the vehicle through which they become real in everyday life.
>
> (Dilworth-Anderson and Cohen 2009: 488–9)

According to Dilworth-Anderson and Cohen (2009), it is important for theorists to examine their own values, assumptions, and history and the influence of these on their approaches to understanding diverse cultural groups. These authors (2009: 489) suggest that examination of one's own background and experiences, including values, may be necessary in studying culturally diverse groups. They conclude that this examination "may lead to understanding the limitations of existing theoretical paradigms and traditions, which shape how groups are approached at many levels."

Social Inequality

It is also necessary to understand the effects of physiological changes, psychological well-being, health status, social class, gender, sexual orientation, and race as they intersect and alter the social realities of older adults and their families (Hooyman and Kiyak 2011). We know that social circumstances early in life can have effects on people that last a lifetime. Experiences related to inequality, oppression, and privilege are experienced within cultural contexts and are powerful determinants of quality of life in later adulthood.

Essential considerations when focusing on diversity of experiences in later adulthood are the lifelong effects of structures of inequality that are institutionalized manifestations of prejudice and discrimination. For many people, the cumulative effects jeopardize the potential of living to old age and, if old age is reached, the quality of life in later adulthood. For example, health status in later adulthood is greatly affected by accessibility and quality of information and services available to meet health care needs throughout one's lifetime, and we know that availability differs within nations and internationally.

Andersen and Collins' (2007: 7) conceptualization of a "matrix of domination model" is useful for understanding experiences related to difference, diversity, and multiculturalism and has implications for study of diversity and aging. They differentiate their theoretical model from a "difference model" that is more likely to focus on the unique experiences of a group of people. While shared experiences related to race, class, and gender are addressed in the difference model, the matrix of domination relational model takes the comparative model a step further and addresses structural relationships between different group experiences. Andersen and Collins (2007: 7–8) write that:

> Thus, when you think relationally, you see the social structures that *simultaneously* generate unique group histories and link them together in society. You then untangle the workings of social systems that shape the experiences of different people and groups, and you move beyond just comparing (for example) gender oppression with race oppression or the oppression of gays and lesbians with that of racial groups. When you recognize the systems of power that mark different groups' experiences, you then possess the conceptual apparatus to think about changing the system, not just documenting the effects of the system on different people.

A global goal: "active ageing"

Maltreatment perpetrated through oppressive systems diminishes individuals' potential for "active ageing." "Active ageing" is defined by the World Health Organization (WHO) as "the process of optimizing opportunities for health, participation, and security in order to enhance quality of life as people age" (WHO 2002: 2). It refers to both individuals and population groups, and an active ageing approach shifts strategic planning to a rights-based approach instead of a needs-based approach because it recognizes the rights of older people to equality of treatment and opportunity. It supports their responsibility to participate in aspects of community life including participation in the political process. The active ageing approach recognizes the importance of diversity of experiences because it regards quality of life to be "an individual's perception of his or her position in life in the context of the culture and value system where they live, and in relation to their goals, expectations, standards and concerns" (WHO 2002: 13).

Determinants over the life course that influence achievement of "active ageing" include: (1) behavioral determinants conducive to healthy lifestyles; (2) determinants related to the physical environment that are supportive of safety and independence and dependence; (3) determinants in the social environment that include "social support, freedom from violence and abuse, and access to lifelong learning;" (4) economic determinants including "income security and access to work throughout the lifecourse as well as social protection;" and (5) health and social services throughout the lifecourse that are "integrated, coordinated, cost-effective, and based on the principle of universal access." Also related to health and social services, WHO supports availability of a "continuum of care from preventive, curative, rehabilitative, long-term to palliative," training in geriatrics and gerontology, and caregiver supports as conducive to active aging. The Active Ageing Policy Framework guided by the United Nations Principles for Older People requires action in the areas of health, participation, and security, and together with the UN International Plan of Action on Ageing provides a map for developing aging policies to improve the health and welfare of older adults (Kalache et al. 2005: 42–3).

Chapter descriptions

Exploration of contemporary theoretical perspectives about aging begins in Chapter 2 with historical information about the development of the multidisciplinary field of gerontology, issues regarding gerontological theorizing and diversity of experiences in aging, and an historical introduction to the development of sociological theories of aging. In Chapter 3, the phenomenological perspective in gerontological theorizing in sociology and narrative gerontology as an example of a phenomenological approach to theory development are presented. In addition to describing basic theoretical concepts, examples of work by researchers addressing diversity of experiences in aging from this perspective are provided.

Chapter 4 explains critical perspectives in gerontological theorizing and provides examples of work by researchers addressing diversity of experiences in aging from the perspective of critical theory. In Chapter 5, feminist perspectives in gerontological theorizing are described, accompanied by examples of aging experiences informed by this perspective's emphasis on the significance of gender in aging.

The life course perspective, explained in Chapter 6, is an important approach for identifying experiences throughout the life course, including accumulation of disadvantage or privilege, that affect quality of life for older individuals. Perspectives on inequality theory and the life course are presented. Chapter 7 explains gerotranscendence theory and provides examples to increase understanding of aging experiences from this perspective.

In Chapter 8, "Theory, Diversity, and Policy," perspectives regarding existing policies and directions for aging policy development are described. Important institutional areas of policy development are identified with attention to the importance of cultural considerations. Global advocacy for policies for the well-being of older people is addressed. Chapter 9 concludes the book with a summary of major themes in aging theory development and implications of the content of this book for developing aging theory, research, and policy.

Summary

Theorizing involves development of ideas that facilitate prediction and understanding and explanation of empirical observations. Sociological theories aid understanding of aging experiences of diverse older adults and their families, communities, and societies as they experience social changes resulting from current demographic realities. Perspectives and theories that will be discussed extensively in this book are phenomenological, critical, feminist, life course, and gerotranscendence approaches to understanding aging and social change. Theories addressing policy perspectives are also included, in addition to policy initiatives to address global needs related to aging populations.

Global demographic changes are resulting in challenges and benefits for societies and people of all ages. Changes include demographic transition, an increasingly rapid process that occurs when increased life expectancy and declining fertility rates drive population aging in a nation. Because people age in different environments, there are variations in social, physical, psychological, and spiritual experiences related to aging. Experiences related to inequality, oppression, and privilege take place within cultural contexts and are powerful determinants of quality of life in later adulthood. Cohort differences, such as changes in women's roles, contribute to diversity of experiences of older adults and introduce new challenges and benefits for families and communities over time. A contemporary perspective, "active ageing," developed by the World Health Organization (WHO), emphasizes the right of older people to continued participation in social institutions and the importance of enhancing quality of life as people age by optimizing opportunities in the areas of health, participation, and security.

2 Development of gerontology and sociological theories of aging

Key concepts

1. Old age has been a topic of study and reflection for thousands of years, but changing social environments, individual and group experiences require continued exploration.
2. Since 1960, research and education about social and behavioral aspects of aging have burgeoned in the new discipline of gerontology and in anthropology, economics, social history, sociology, cognitive and developmental psychologies, and social work.
3. Social aging refers to the nature of the society in which aging occurs, the influence that society has on its aging individuals, and the impact aging individuals have on their society.
4. Many social gerontological theories exist, but there are conflicts about the lack of a general theory that can become an organizing framework for understanding and explaining aging.
5. Differences among and within social science fields contribute to controversies about approaches for developing gerontological knowledge, but concepts in diverse approaches are the building blocks of theory although objectives and methods are different.
6. Interests of social gerontologists that are of particular interest to sociologists include, but are not limited to, the process of creation and change in social organizations as they respond to age-related experiences associated with birth, socialization, role transitions, retirement, and death.
7. New problems of societal aging include extension of the life course, changes in the age structures of nations, changes in family structures and relationships, and changes in governmental expectations and responsibilities.
8. Responses of labor markets, political institutions, retirement and pension systems, and healthcare organizations to issues pertaining to age need to be explained.
9. Irving Rosow's conceptualization of role theory proposed that roles of older adults are socially unstructured because they do not have a specific age role and their social position is determined by the loss of major responsibility and authority.

10. James Dowd applied exchange theory to the experiences of older people in industrializing societies and proposed that they will experience decreased social interaction because others will experience fewer rewards in relating to them, and he predicted that policies such as mandatory retirement would prevail.
11. It became apparent in the 1970s that there were countervailing influences, and in the U.S. older people began to influence aging policy on their own behalf with the result that workplace policies requiring retirement because of age became illegal for most positions.
12. Early theories of aging often assumed that age was a "leveler," that people became more similar as they aged, and failed to address attributes such as race, ethnicity, gender, sexual orientation, disability status, social class, immigration status, and nationality that continue to affect individuals and groups as they become older.
13. In 1998, John Rowe and Robert Kahn published findings from an eight-year research study that focused on what it means to age successfully, and they believed that prior to this study researchers in the field of aging were preoccupied with disease, disability, and chronological age and failed to adequately consider psychosocial influences on well-being of older adults.
14. An example of the relationship between theory and research exists in Robert Atchley's experience of formulating retirement theory that was followed by research about adult development, aging, and adaptation during the retirement transition, which was followed by formulation of theoretical implications based on the research findings.

Introduction

Chapter 2 provides information about historical views of aging, contemporary development of gerontological study, issues in development of social gerontological theories, and introduction to sociological perspectives and their relationship to diversity of aging experiences.

Foundations of gerontological study

Old age has been a topic of study and reflection for thousands of years, but changing social environments, individual, and group experiences require continued exploration. Perceptions of old age have varied tremendously and reflect diverse social contexts and individual experiences. The philosopher and poet Ptah-hotep, writing in Egypt in 2500 BCE, provided a despairing view of old age as a time of cognitive loss and physical weakness and pain. While bodily decline became a universally recurring theme throughout the world, in the East in ancient times older people thrived. Cultural contexts were important determinants of aging experiences, the well-being of older people was supported in Confucian and Taoist principles (Achenbaum 2005). In the Quran, the reality of physical decline associated with aging was considered a sign of Allah's power (Thursby 2000: 159).

Confucianism supported the well-being of older people in its principles about relations between superiors and inferiors. In his chronological view of moral development, Confucius posited aging as beneficial when he wrote "At fifteen, I applied myself to wisdom; at thirty, I grew stronger at it; at forty I no longer had doubts; at sixty there was nothing on earth that could shake me; at seventy I could follow the dictates of my heart without disobeying the moral law" (Thang 2000: 196). For centuries, members of Chinese families owed strict obedience to the oldest man, and older women prevailed over sons and daughters on the basis of age (Achenbaum 2005: 21).

Ancient Western civilizations held diverse views of old age. In ancient Greece, Hippocrates catalogued specific illnesses of old age, yet beginning in the seventh century BC Sparta was ruled by a council of men, the *gerousia*, who were at least 60 years old and selected for their wisdom. In ancient Rome, Virgil (70–19 BC) and Juvenal (60–130 AD) lamented old age, but Cicero (106–43 BC) considered experience to be an advantage of aging while he also acknowledged negative aspects. He wrote in *De senectute* that:

> It is not by muscle, speed, or physical dexterity that great things are achieved, but by reflection, force of character, and judgment; in these qualities, old age is usually not poorer, but is even richer...old age, so far from being feeble and inactive, is ever busy and doing and effecting something.
>
> (Falconer 1923: 27, 35, in Achenbaum 2005: 22)

Hebrew scripture also provides diverse views of aging, including gruesome descriptions of physical decline while elsewhere commanding respect for elders and celebrating longevity as a reward for faithfulness to God. According to Achenbaum (2005), emphasis in most traditions on physical changes occurring with aging resulted in a widespread tendency to associate aging with disease and death even though positive attributes were also identified.

Contemporary development of gerontological study

Since the 1940s, professional interest in the problems of older people has been evident in the development of interdisciplinary organizations and conferences including the American Society on Aging, Gerontological Society of America, International Congress of Gerontology, International Federation on Ageing, the United Nations NGO (nongovernmental organization) Committee on Ageing, and annual programs recognizing the United Nations International Day of Older Persons established in 1990. Since 1960, research and education about social and behavioral aspects of aging have burgeoned in the new discipline of gerontology and in anthropology, economics, social history, sociology, and cognitive and developmental psychologies, and social work. Gerontological interest is evident in university courses and specializations in many disciplines, including sociology, and development of gerontology departments and research institutes within and outside of other university departments. Journals and books about aspects of aging have been published in many languages about diverse topics. Often the process of aging is studied as part of the life course with attention to the fact that there are variations in aging experiences and cultural contexts.

Consistent with the historical emphasis on physical decline, in 1903 the term "gerontology" was initially used by Elie Metchnikoff, who believed that aging was the result of "intestinal putrefaction" (Birren 1999: 460). The term "geriatrics" is more often used in medicine and other health care fields. Over a century later, gerontology encompasses a greatly expanded sphere of knowledge and inquiry including multidisciplinary academic and practice interests. In reality, *"Aging is neither predictably positive nor predictably negative.* For some people it is mainly positive, for others it is mainly negative, and for still others it is somewhere in between" (Atchley and Barusch 2004: 5).

In its "use of reason to understand aging" gerontology addresses physical, psychological, social psychological, and social aspects of human development, and gerontological study encompasses many academic and practice disciplines (Atchley and Barusch 2004: 3). Defining itself as a science, gerontology has expanded from its initial emphasis on biology and biomedicine, psychology, and the social sciences to include anthropology, demography, economics, epidemiology, history, humanities and arts, political science, social work, and other professions assisting older people (Bengtson et al. 2005).

The three areas focused upon by gerontologists include the aged, aging as a developmental process, and age as it relates to structure and behavior within species (Bengtson et al. 2005). The primary components of gerontology include:

> The study of physical aging examines the causes and consequences of the body's declining capacity to renew itself; the physical effects of bodily aging; and the means for preventing, treating, or compensating for illness or disability caused by or related to physical aging.
>
> The study of psychological aging focuses on the effects of aging on sensory processes, perception, coordination, mental capacity, human development, personality, and coping ability.
>
> Social psychological aging looks at the interaction of the individual with his or her environment and includes such topics as attitudes, values, beliefs, social roles, self-image, and adjustment to aging.
>
> Social aging refers to the nature of the society in which aging occurs, the influence that society has on its aging individuals, and the impact aging individuals have on their society.
>
> (Atchley and Barusch 2004: 3)

Sociological study of aging is one component of social gerontology, the area of gerontology addressing nonphysical aspects of aging. Since social gerontology focuses on the study of individual aging and the relationship between aging and society, physical aging is of interest to social gerontologists only with regard to its influence on adaptation of individuals and societies to each other. In a new development in the 1940s, some social scientists began to study normal, healthy older people. Prior to this time, research about later adulthood focused on hospitalized or institutionalized people (Atchley and Barusch 2004). In 1955, the Duke Longitudinal Studies began to explore "normal," or normative, aging. The researchers wanted to learn about diverse experiences in later adulthood that were not caused by disease (Busse and Maddox 1985).

Social gerontology has its own unique theoretical perspectives, concepts, and research interests in addition to perspectives and concepts that it shares with other social sciences. Commonly used terms in sociology and other social sciences may be used differently in gerontological study. Atchley and Barusch (2004) provide an example of the concept of "self" which is frequently used in social sciences to refer to "ideas about oneself that are developed in interaction with others…. However, in gerontology we much more often study people whose self-concept is already well-developed and not very sensitive to outside influence…. Within gerontology, we are much more likely to explore how individuals *enhance, maintain,* or *defend* their self-concepts than how their self-concepts are initially established." Furthermore, social gerontology's information about aging tends to be more extensive than aging content generally in the social sciences (Atchley and Barusch 2004: 10).

Attention to gerontological theories and theory development has been inconsistent over the past 70 years. During the 1940s, the field of biology devoted considerable attention to homeostatic mechanisms and aging, and in the 1950s psychologists explored linkages between early and later phases of human development, especially cognition, with a similar level of interest. Considerable activity ensued in the 1960s with debates among social gerontologists about disengagement theory, activity theory, subcultural theory, and role theory.

There was a resurgence of interest in development of aging theory during the 1990s. This was reflected in articles about disengagement theory published in *The Gerontologist* (published by the Gerontological Society of America), symposia on theory development presented at the Annual Meetings of the American Sociological Association, and papers about a wide variety of theoretical models that were presented at the 1993 International Congress of Gerontology and published in the *Canadian Journal of Aging* in 1995 (Bengtson et al.1996).

Books devoted to explication of theories in several disciplines include *Emergent Theories of Aging* (1988), edited by Birren and Bengtson; *Handbook of Theories of Aging* (1999), edited by Bengtson and Schaie; and *Handbook of Theories of Aging,* 2nd edition (2009), edited by Bengtson et al. While these books include broad theoretical perspectives, *The Cambridge Handbook of Age and Ageing* (2005), edited by M.L. Johnson, generally addresses issues of theoretical interest from narrower topically oriented perspectives. The current volume, *Understanding Aging and Diversity: Theories and Concepts,* adds to the professional literature about theories of aging by providing a compendium of contemporary gerontological theories in the field of sociology and addressing the relevance of these perspectives to studies that facilitate understanding of diversity of experiences in later adulthood.

Issues in development of social gerontological theories

Impediments and differences in gerontological theories and theorizing

Social gerontology includes many theories even though this field has been described as lacking in theories. Some gerontologists have considered the field to be data-rich and theory-poor (Birren 1999; Settersten and Dobransky 2000). In reality, many social gerontological theories exist, as will be demonstrated in this book, but there are conflicts about the lack of a general theory that can become an organizing framework for understanding and explaining aging. Opinions differ about whether an overarching theory is necessary, or even possible. Efforts have been made to develop theories of this type, including disengagement theory and activity theory, but these were discredited because of their failure to adequately address diversity in aging experiences.

According to Atchley (1999: vii), dilemmas about development of gerontological theories may result from the reality that "its journals are filled with research reports that are best described as abstracted empiricism, loaded with descriptions and statements of relation tied to empirical measures rather than to interconnected theoretical constructs that constitute full-fledged theory." Nevertheless, as Atchley indicated in 1999, there were already theories of aging in many disciplines, and these addressed varied topics, including stages of adult development (Erikson 1963; Erikson 1997; Levinson 1990); stress and coping in later life (Pearlin 1991); caregiving stress (Kinney et al. 1995; Biegel and Blum 1990); social isolation in old age (Kuypers and Bengtson 1973); adaptation to role loss (Cumming and Henry 1961; Havighurst 1963; Rosow 1976); and the life course (Atchley 1975; Riley 1994).

Bengtson et al. (2005: 4) have identified five impediments to theoretical progress in gerontology:

> (1) the inability or unwillingness to integrate theory-based knowledge within topic areas and synthesize theoretical insights into the context of existing knowledge; (2) the difficulty of crossing disciplinary boundaries in order to create multidisciplinary explanations and interpretations of phenomena of ageing; (3) the strong 'problem-solving' orientation of gerontology that tends to detract from basic research programs where theory plays a central role; (4) the trend toward focusing on individuals in micro settings while ignoring wider social contexts, which tends to dampen even middle-range theory building (Hagestad and Dannefer, 2001); (5) epistemological debates over the virtues of the scientific approach to knowledge or whether human behavior can be understood at all in terms of laws, causes and prediction (mirroring theoretical disagreements within sociology since the mid-1960s).

Differences among and within social science fields contribute to controversies about approaches for developing gerontological knowledge. However, concepts in diverse approaches are the building blocks of theory although objectives and methods are different. Positivism continues to predominate in mainstream gerontological research and uses the traditional definition of scientific theory as:

> a deductive one, starting with definitions of general concepts and putting forward a number of logically ordered propositions about the relationships among concepts. Concepts are linked to empirical phenomena through operational definitions, from which hypotheses are derived and then tested against empirical observations. A general theory allows investigators to deduce logically a number of quite specific statements, or explanations, about the nature and behavior of a large class of phenomena.
>
> (Bengtson et al. 2005: 7-8)

An approach for developing aging theory that is different from the traditional scientific approach uses inductive or "grounded" theoretical approaches and qualitative methods in efforts to explain aging phenomena. This approach begins with the data and leads to identification of key concepts and their relationship to each another (Bengtson et al. 2005: 7). Proponents advocate for a more interpretive perspective. According to Bengtson et al. (2005: 7):

> They [proponents] argue that general explanatory arguments are likely to miss so much of people's experiences that they are seriously flawed and inadequate. Researchers in these traditions focus on describing and understanding how social interactions proceed, and on the subjective meanings of age and ageing phenomena. Knowledge of the social world derives from the meanings individuals attach to their social situations. A "theory"– many social constructionists prefer the term "sensitizing scheme"–is useful to the extent that it provides a deeper understanding of particular social events and settings (Gubrium and Holstein, 1999). The interpretive perspective is premised on the notion that individuals are active agents and can change the nature of their social environments. Thus there cannot be general theories of ageing reflecting 'immutable laws' of human social organization (Turner, 2003).

Bengtson et al. (2005: 7) identify five major types of differences in contemporary gerontological theories:

(1) their underlying assumptions (particularly about human nature – whether human behavior is essentially determined and thus predictable – or whether individuals are essentially creative and agentic);
(2) their subject matter (reflecting specific disciplinary interests, or whether the focus is on macrolevel institutions or on microlevel personal encounters and interactions);
(3) their epistemological approach (positivistic, interpretive, or critical);

(4) their methodological approach (deductive or inductive); and
(5) their ultimate objectives (whether they aim largely at describing things, explaining or even predicting them, or changing the way things are).

Epistomological issues: variations in classification of theories

How do gerontologists organize what they know about theory? In social gerontology, there are debates about forms of knowledge and use of theory that gerontologists believe need to be addressed through epistemology, or identification of *"how we know what we think we know"* (Bengtson et al. 2005: 3). Victor Marshall (1999: 435) points out that "Doing theory well requires a broadly based and deeply historically textured sense of the field, and it involves processes of comparing and contrasting theoretical approaches." According to Marshall, classifications of social theories of aging are not always in agreement, and he suggests that approaches for making connections between theoretical approaches include: (1) theoretical contrast and conflict; (2) typology as an approach to understanding theory; and (3) telling stories and making connections as an approach to understanding theory. Contrast and conflict were apparent in development of activity theory as an alternative to Cumming and Henry's (1961) formulation of disengagement theory. Likewise, Marshall and Tindale (1978) contrasted their political economy approach with mainstream sociology with its normative assumptions (Marshall 1999: 434, 436, 437).

Focusing on the second classificatory approach, Marshall (1999: 437–8) developed a typology with two dimensions of contrast. His typology cross-classifies normative, bridging, and interpretive levels of theoretical analysis with macro, linking, and micro levels of theoretical analysis. The following list includes the theoretical perspectives specified in Marshall's (1999: 437–8) typology and their dual classifications:

- Macro/Normative: structuralism, modernization, aging theory
- Macro/Bridging: interest group theory, institutional theory
- Macro/Interpretive: political economy
- Linking/Normative: disengagement, activity, birth and fortune thesis, age stratification
- Linking/Bridging: life course perspective, feminist theories
- Linking/Interpretive: critical theory, symbolic interactionism and phenomenology, cultural anthropology
- Micro/Normative: role theory, developmental theory, conventional economic and rational choice theory
- Micro/Bridging: exchange theory
- Micro/Interpretive: self and identity theories including continuity theory, career/status passage, dramaturgical theory.

For his third approach, Marshall (1999: 441) recommends "telling stories and making connections" through individual linkages or other historical connections to people who developed or worked on the theories. In this way, a "more human face" can be placed on theory and theorists. In "Analyzing Social Theories of Aging" (1999: 448–9), Marshall provides examples of different generational stories about theories of aging and concludes:

> We have, then, three different generational stories about sociological theories of aging, developed by Hendricks [1992], Bengtson and colleagues [1996, 1997], and the Lynotts [1996]; these stories are not wholly consistent, yet each challenges us to think in new ways about theoretical continuity and change. Bengtson, Burgess, and Parrott (1997) emphasize an important point, that understanding or discovery of a phenomena is seldom achieved by the solo investigator, but rather is a social process within a community of investigators involving discussion and criticism between new and previous findings and explanations' (pS84). Theories help to organize observations that are pooled by the community of scientists within theory groups, and it thereby helps these observations to be seen as either consistent with existing theory or anomalous. 'These anomalities (and their emergent explanations) are the basis for 'paradigm shifts' and 'scientific revolutions' which can leapfrog the progress of knowledge forward (Kuhn, 1962)' (Bengtson et al. 1997, p. S84)....
>
> One of the giants in our field, Bernice Neugarten [1964, 1965, 1970, 1987], has successively embraced and advocated a number of theoretical positions, beginning with developmental psychology in her early work and in some of her work on the Kansas City Studies of Aging. She then turned to a very deterministic, structural-functionalist perspective when she emphasized the power of normative determination in shaping age-appropriate behavior and later advocated an interpretive theoretical approach that emphasizes the capacity for choice and human agency.

Considerations in developing sociological theories of aging

Interests of social gerontologists that are of particular interest to sociologists include, but are not limited to, the process of change in social organizations as they respond to socialization, role transitions, or death. New problems pertaining to societal aging include changes in family structures and relationships and changes in governmental expectations and responsibilities. Phenomena to be explained include responses of institutions such as labor markets, healthcare organizations, retirement and pension systems, and political institutions to changing age demographics.

The 1970s: influences of time, place, and predisposing sociological orientations

The importance of recognition and acknowledgment of the influences of time, place, and predisposing sociological orientations on theoretical conceptualizations about aging is exemplified in the theories of functionalists Irving Rosow and James Dowd published during the 1970s in the United States. Addressing experiences of older people within a developing capitalistic economy, they suggested that economic changes have a preeminent role in marginalization of older people. Typical of early sociological theories of aging, implications of diversity related to characteristics such as race, ethnicity, sexual orientation, and gender were not addressed.

In his application of role theory to aging, Rosow theorized that older workers become obsolete due to rapidly changing technology. He suggested that as a consequence, they experience role loss due to devaluation and exclusion from significant social participation, and systematic status loss occurs for an entire cohort. According to Rosow, the lives of older people are socially unstructured because they do not have a specific age role and are not socialized "to the fate of aging." Therefore the loss of major responsibility and authority determines their social position. Rosow suggested that efforts that support the social context would be more effective than direct service programs because there is greater flexibility in informal roles. Therefore, he advised that social policy should aim to optimize naturally occurring social forces that support spontaneous relationships, voluntary groups, and informal as opposed to formal roles (Rosow 1976: 465, 469).

Dowd applied exchange theory to the experiences of older people in industrializing societies. Influenced by George Homans's proposition that profit from social or economic exchange is equal to rewards minus costs, Dowd proposed that decisions regarding interaction with older people are influenced by other peoples' perception of the value of the exchange with an older person. He suggested that interaction is more likely to continue if it is rewarding and that older people will experience decreased social interaction because others will experience fewer rewards in relating to them. Therefore the relative power of older people will decrease in their social relationships. According to Dowd, decreased social interaction of older people in the U.S. occurs partly because of impaired health, reduced income, and loss of a spouse. According to this theory, increased specialization of knowledge since the Industrial Revolution and cohort-defining levels of education, socioeconomic status of the family of origin, and occupational aspirations jeopardized the status of older people, and mandatory retirement was an inevitable outcome. Dowd regarded implementation of mandatory retirement policies by the federal government to be an exchange of leisure time for older people for workforce positions for younger people (Dowd 1975: 586–8).

Regardless of the belief of some sociologists that policies such as mandatory retirement based on age rather than employee qualifications would prevail, it became apparent in the 1970s that there were countervailing influences. In the U.S., older people began to influence aging policy on their own behalf. Joined by allies including human service professionals, academics, community organization leaders, clergy, and legislators in their efforts to challenge ageist practices, older people and their collaborators succeeded in achieving revocation of federal and state regulations supporting mandatory retirement based on age for most employment positions in the U.S. The founder of the Gray Panthers organization,

Maggie Kuhn, responded to losing her employment due to mandatory retirement policies by establishing this advocacy organization that provided structure for a broad range of civil rights advocacy efforts, including opposition to mandatory retirement policies.

An additional sociological theory of aging from the 1970s, Kuypers and Bengtson's (1973) social reconstruction theory, posits negative effects of modernization on the lives of older people, but it also proposes approaches for opposing these effects. According to Kuypers and Bengtson (1973: 182), in social breakdown syndrome "an individual's sense of self, his ability to mediate between self and society, and his orientation to personal mastery are functions of the kind of *social labeling* and valuing that he experiences in aging." Providing an example of multidisciplinary influences on theoretical development, in this case a relationship between psychological and sociological theories, this systems perspective drew upon the formulation of social breakdown syndrome by Gruenberg and Zusman (1964) and Zusman (1966) that was intended to explain negative psychological functioning in the general population (Kuypers and Bengtson 1973). Kuypers and Bengtson (1973) argued that older people are likely to be susceptible to social labeling because of social reorganization in later adulthood. They believed that social reorganization took place in later life because as aging occurs social conditions such as lack of reference groups, role loss, and inappropriate or vague normative information deprive individuals of feedback about identification, appropriate roles and behavior, and individual value in their social world. Lack of feedback was believed to create vulnerability to, and dependence on, external sources of labeling that communicate that the older adult is useless and obsolete and results in social breakdown. Systemic changes including shrinking roles, loss of normative guidance, and lack of appropriate reference groups were identified as increasing the vulnerability of older people. Successful role performance, adaptive capacity and personal feelings of mastery and inner control were considered types of competence that suffer in the breakdown cycle.

In spite of this negative view of systemic influences on aging experiences, Kuypers and Bengtson described responses that were more consistent with those of Maggie Kuhn and the Gray Panthers than Rosow and Dowd's proposed responses. Kuypers and Bengtson (1973) indicated that it is important to try to liberate older people from the view that worth is contingent on economic roles. They proposed that adaptive capacity could be enhanced by reducing poor health, poverty, and substandard housing and that personal strengths could be facilitated by enabling internal locus of control. Self-determination and control of policy and administration were considered foundations for competent aging.

Successful aging: the MacArthur Foundation study

In 1998, John Rowe and Robert Kahn published findings from an eight-year research study that focused on what it means to age successfully, what individuals can do to achieve this, and what changes would enable people to live more successfully in the United States. They believed that prior to this study researchers in the field of aging were preoccupied with disease, disability, and chronological age and failed to adequately consider psychosocial influences on well-being of older adults. Their research was rooted in Rowe and Kahn's interest in factors that allowed individuals to have good physical and mental functioning in old age. Their study focused on over one thousand high functioning older people in the U.S. and hundreds of pairs of Swedish twins (Rowe and Kahn 1998).

Rowe and Kahn believed that this study contributed to a reorientation toward a "successful aging" theme in gerontology. They concluded that six familiar myths about older adults were refuted by the research findings: "to be old is to be sick," "you can't teach an old dog new tricks," "the horse is out of the barn," "the secret to successful aging is to choose your parents wisely," "the lights many be on but the voltage is low," and "the elderly don't pull their own weight." They were referring to realities that in the U.S. chronic illnesses are more prevalent than acute, infectious diseases, as well as the finding that old people can and do learn new things. Findings also indicated that risk reduction and health promotion is possible in old age, and functioning may even increase beyond an individual's prior level; genes and aging are connected but the significance of genetics is overstated; sexual activity varies greatly in old age, with cultural norms, health or illness, and availability of a partner the most significant variables; and older workers bring increased insight and experience to their place of employment and often meet or surpass expectations. Rowe and Kahn concluded that the findings indicate that people can experience "successful aging," and personality and lifestyle factors can be identified that can increase the chances of "successful aging." They noted the importance of social factors, remarking that "we can have a dramatic impact on our own success or failure in aging" but that what people can do for themselves depends to some extent on social policies, as well as attitudes and expectations regarding older adults (Rowe and Kahn 1998: 18).

Robert Atchley: continuity theory: example of analytical process from theory to research to theory development

Sociologists have developed important theoretical perspectives that have led to research, and research findings have been the basis for formulating additional theories of aging. This process creates growth of knowledge in social gerontology. Robert Atchley's (1999) development of theories followed by research about adult development, aging, and adaptation during the retirement transition, and his formulation of theoretical implications based on research findings provides an example of this process of knowledge building.

In his Preface to *Continuity and Adaptation in Aging: Creating Positive Experiences* (1999: viii), Atchley provides insight into his longstanding interests in people's adaptation to changes related to aging. Developing his interest in gerontology during the 1960s when the field was searching for an orienting framework and embroiled in controversies regarding disengagement and activity theories, he began his dissertation in the 1960s about the influence of retirement on women's self-concepts. Atchley (1999: ix) developed hypotheses predicting "negative effects for the self when women retired and thus no longer had a work identity." He continues by describing findings contrary to his expectations:

> But as I was pretesting my interview schedule, I was brought up short by a woman who, at the end of a pretest interview said, "is that it? When are you going to ask me about the good stuff about retirement?" I realized that I had unconsciously biased the interview by asking only about areas where negative effects of retirement might be expected. Using focus groups of retired women, I developed a more balanced set of questions.
>
> I was thoroughly impressed with the positive adjustment I found among both retired women schoolteachers and retired women telephone operators....None of the negative effects I expected materialized because these women carried their occupational identities with them into retirement and continued to derive self-esteem from them.
>
> (Atchley 1999: ix)

Atchley (1999) conducted a study in 1968 that included over 4,000 retired teachers and telephone company employees of both genders and found that an overwhelming majority had adjusted well to retirement, continued to possess their occupational identities, and had high self-esteem. Women and men adapted to retirement equally well although the findings indicated gender differences in other areas. Atchley's results led to a preliminary statement of a theory of identity continuity.

Subsequent to developing his statement of identity continuity, Atchley began a longitudinal research study of retirement of females and males that continued from 1975 to 1995, the Ohio Longitudinal Study of Aging and Adaptation (OLSAA), in a small town in Ohio. This study was influenced by Atchley's (1999: xi–xii) interest in newfound multidisciplinary "theoretical strands" that he considered complementary, including Buckley's (1967) feedback systems theory, Riegel's (1976) dialectical theory of continuous adult development, Erikson's (1963) cumulative stage theory, and Kelly's (1955) personal construct theory.

At the conclusion of the OLSAA research, 300 respondents from the initial sample of over 1,000 people age 50 and over remained as participants. Data was collected on subjects including external social frameworks that made up their lifestyle, marital status, number of children, occupation, employment status, leisure activities, community involvement, involvement with family and friends, health and disability, financial resources, religious affiliation, and retirement. Atchley was able to formulate new theories during the course of the research, including theories that were not anticipated at the inception of the study.

Atchley (1999) found that the overwhelming majority of people in the research sample adapted well to positive and negative changes in their lives. Areas of continuity, stability, and discontinuity were identified over time as participants responded to a wide range of physical and psychological changes and shifts in social roles and support networks. He theorized that continuity is the most prevalent form of adaptation, that continuity and change can exist simultaneously, and that it is important to achieve balance between these at various times. Atchley theorized that continuity can occur when there are no changes or, alternatively, when there are minor changes within general patterns. He considered discontinuity to occur when there are dramatic shifts that may involve significant departures from past patterns. Atchley had begun with theory development, conducted research based on his theorizing, and developed new theories about continuity and discontinuity in later adulthood based on research findings.

Summary

This chapter describes historical and theoretical developments that provide a foundation for learning about contemporary sociological theories addressed in the following chapters. Old age has been studied for thousands of years, but global social changes create the need for continued exploration. Contemporary gerontological study began to develop in the mid-1900s as people recognized that life expectancy in developed nations had increased substantially at the same time as increased industrialization and modernization affected multiple institutional areas.

Sociological study of aging is within the purview of social aging, and social aging refers to the nature of the society in which aging occurs, the influence that society has on its aging individuals, and the impact aging individuals have on their society. Social issues that are addressed include increased life expectancy, changes in family structures and relationships, and changes in governmental roles. Sociologist Robert Atchley's research about aging and retirement experiences illustrates a process of development of theory with implications for research studies followed by research with implications for theory development.

Time, place, sociological orientation, and personal biases can influence development of sociological theories of aging, and theories reflect different approaches to theory development and research. Early theories of aging often assumed that age was a "leveler," that people became more similar as they aged, and failed to address attributes such as race, ethnicity, gender, sexual orientation, disability status, social class, immigration status, and nationality that continue to affect individuals and groups as they become older. Continuity theory and theories of successful aging have given greater consideration to diversity of experiences in aging. Consideration of additional theories in the following chapters will include discussion of ways that theoretical perspectives, theories, and research informed by theory can increase understanding of diversity of experiences in later adulthood.

Many social gerontological theories exist, but there are conflicts about the lack of a general theory that can become an organizing framework for understanding and explaining aging. Opinions differ about whether an overarching theory is necessary or possible. Disengagement theory, activity theory, role theory, and exchange theory are examples of efforts to develop overarching theories.

3   Phenomenological gerontology

Key concepts

1. The foundation of social phenomenology is in the work of European philosophers Edmund Husserl, Martin Heidegger, Gabriel Marcel, Simone de Beauvoir, Maurice Merleau-Ponty, and Jean-Paul Sartre.
2. Phenomenology has continued to be influenced by Husserl's belief that the phenomenologist suspends belief in the existence of the outer world, things within it, and validity of statements about the world for his analytical purpose. Belief is suspended, in order to refrain intentionally and systematically from all judgments related to the existence of the outer world.
3. Phenomenology was brought to the United States by sociologist Alfred Schutz during the 1930s, and his emphasis on the social construction of reality influenced development of social phenomenology.
4. Schutz connected Husserl's conceptualization of phenomenology to Max Weber's conceptualization of the ideal type, and this contributed to Schutz's formulation of phenomenological analysis.
5. Processes that he considered to be first-order typifications in which a shared social world is constructed as people bring together enduring and typical experiences create the basis of second-order typifications that are rational intellectual models of the social world based on the first-order typifications.
6. The use of phenomenological approaches in aging studies contrasts starkly with the biomedical model that focuses primarily on bodily failures.
7. Phenomenological gerontology theorizes that knowledge that is useful for developing phenomenological understanding is available in narratives provided by older people.
8. Jaber Gubrium and James Holstein's phenomenological gerontological theorizing focuses on exploration of ordinary ways that older people from diverse backgrounds experience daily life, manage successes and failures, and construct their past and future in relation to the present.
9. Gubrium and Holstein believe that individual meanings of old age are connected to continuing aspects of a person's biography that make it possible for affirmative construction of later life.

10. The reality that older adults engage in metatheorizing as reflection on their activities is a key aspect of phenomenological gerontology, and narrative construction is viewed as dynamic so that interpretation of one's own experiences can change over time through individuals' ordinary theorizing.

11. Narrative gerontology is an approach to understanding later adulthood from a phenomenological perspective and is theorized to have a root metaphor with four characteristics: presupposition of an existential-ontological image of human beings as storytellers and storylisteners who are stories; lives and lifestyles are made up of facticity but re-storying can also occur; interrelated dimensions consisting of a structured story, a sociocultural story, interpersonal dimensions, and personal dimensions; and a personal story is to some extent idiosyncratic, unique, and unknowable.

12. Narrative gerontology suggests research topics that include approaches to theory construction in gerontology; elements of the story of theory construction in gerontology, including the influence of lifestories of theorists; the nature of truth from a narrative gerontology perspective; and education and training issues.

Introduction

Chapter 3 provides an introduction to social phenomenology; description of phenomenological gerontology, including narrative gerontology; an example of narrative interpretation in an analysis of interviews in a study of Swedish older people between the ages of 95 and 103; and phenomenological analysis of interviews in two studies in the United States: "Identity Careers of Older Gay Men and Lesbians" and "Narratives of Forgiveness in Old Age."

Foundations of phenomenological study

Precursors of contemporary social phenomenology include the work of German philosopher Edmund Husserl, who developed phenomenology during the 1890s as the systematic investigation of consciousness, and European phenomenologists Martin Heidegger, Gabriel Marcel, Simone de Beauvoir, Maurice Merleau-Ponty, and Jean-Paul Sartre. Husserl's conceptualization of phenomenology strongly influenced Alfred Schutz, who brought phenomenology to the United States in the 1930s. Schutz's work led to variations of interpretive sociology, including reality constructionism and ethnomethodology, and his emphasis on the social construction of reality strongly influenced his students at the New School for Social Research, including Peter Berger, Harold Garfinkel, Thomas Luckmann, and Maurice Nathanson (Longino and Powell 2009).

Schutz was interested in studying people's construction of objects and taken-for-granted knowledge about these. He connected Husserl's conceptualization of phenomenology to Max Weber's conceptualization of the ideal type, and this contributed to Schutz's formulation of phenomenological analysis. He believed that ideal types are continually being constructed and are constantly adjusted and revised based on the observer's direct and indirect experiences. Processes that he considered to be first-order typifications in which a shared social world is constructed as people bring together enduring and typical experiences create the basis of second-order typifications that are rational intellectual models of the social world based on the first-order typifications (Schutz 1967).

According to Schutz, people learn typified meanings for doing common activities. In their search for meaningful involvement with the world, people are attentive to themes, interpretations that provide meanings, and motivations. Internalized typifications tend to become sedimented beneath full awareness, and therefore people assume that their knowledge is objective and shared by everyone else. Despite assumptions of common knowledge, interpretations differ because the uniqueness of each person's biography results in distinctive typifications and recipes for action that are the tools used by the individual's consciousness to construct an arena of human awareness and action (Schutz 1967).

Phenomenology has continued to be influenced by Husserl's belief that the phenomenologist suspends belief in the existence of the outer world, things within it, and validity of statements about the world for his analytical purpose. Belief in its existence is suspended, in order to refrain intentionally and systematically from all judgments related to the existence of the outer world. Husserl referred to this as "putting the world in brackets" or "performing the phenomenological reduction." This is intended to enable the phenomenologist to "go beyond the natural attitude of a man living within the world he accepts, be it reality or mere appearance" (Schutz 1945: 82–3).

Radina, Hennon, and Gibbons (2008: 142) explain a phenomenological framework in the introduction to their phenomenological analysis of divorce and mid- and later-life families:

> Phenomenological understanding highlights how people give meaning to the life they are living, a focus on individual consciousness. Experience is a crucial aspect of living, a consciousness of one's being a physical and psychological person (corporeality) as well as one's relationship to the physical and social world (relationality). It is also how the immediate world is experienced spatially and temporally. Phenomenology scrutinizes and seeks understanding of how people experience and accomplish everyday reality and how it is inter subjectively structured. People's perspectives, voices, meanings, and their lives as experienced by them are prioritized. The focus is on culture and interpretation, bargaining, emergence, and inventiveness. Consistent attention is paid in phenomenological analysis to how individuals give meaning to the objects of their consciousness or experiences... How people construct their identities around such issues as being divorced (e.g., blame, sense of failure or success, freedom, and 'ex') and their relationships with their children, lovers, ex-spouses, and so forth, is considered more important than positive paradigms of explanation. Thus, in employing phenomenology...we are interested in how people 'make sense' of their life

worlds, and their social position as 'divorced' within this world. Direct descriptions of these experiences are sought…The phenomenological approach intends to maintain fidelity to the phenomena of interest within the context of the life as lived and described by the person conscious of and experiencing these phenomena.

Basic concepts in phenomenological gerontology

Phenomenological gerontology provides insights into meanings and subjective sense of self that are important in aging identity. The use of phenomenological approaches in aging studies contrasts starkly with the dominant biomedical model that focuses primarily on bodily failures. Knowledge that is useful for developing phenomenological understanding is available in narratives provided by older people.

Phenomenological gerontology that is consistent with the main tenets of phenomenology has developed from work of Jaber Gubrium and others. Gubrium and Holstein's gerontological theorizing focuses on exploration of "the ordinary ways the elderly experience daily living, how they manage both successes and failures, and on the manner they construct their pasts and futures in relation to present events and developments" (Gubrium and Holstein 2000: 3). Gubrium (2001: 19) values a qualitative approach to studying aging experiences in which the stories that people tell about their lives reveal recognizable experiences and examine "particular sites, occasions, and texts of lived experience to discern in detail how experience is narratively conveyed in the ways it is or otherwise could be." Gerontological phenomenologists study the process of social construction of aging by "bracketing" or placing aside the reality of aging and age-related concepts and focusing on stories told by older people (Lynott and Lynott 1996).

Experiences of change and stability in roles during later adulthood are seen as continuation of lifelong processes, and for some individuals later adulthood is viewed in complex sets of categories that include caregiving, employment, friendship, and other activities rather than specific age categories (Gubrium and Holstein 2000: 1, 4). Historical circumstances, cultural backgrounds, and biographical experiences are considered important, reflecting phenomenological gerontology as an approach that supports study of diversity (Gubrium and Holstein 2003). Gubrium and Holstein (2003: 8, 10) believe that individual meanings of old age are connected to continuing aspects of a person's biography that make it possible for affirmative construction of later life.

Metatheorizing

The reality that older adults engage in metatheorizing as reflection on their activities is a key aspect of phenomenological gerontology. Consistent with a developmental view, narrative construction is dynamic, and interpretation of one's own experiences can change over time through individuals' ordinary theorizing. The material body is subjectively mediated and different from the objective body, and people assign different meanings to their own bodies despite objective bodily conditions.

Cultural and personal expectations influence development of meanings held by individuals (Gergen and Gergen 2000; Gubrium and Holstein 2000). For example, in "Gender, ethnicity, and social relations in the narratives of elderly Sikh men and women" (2006), Mand demonstrates how narratives of older men and women who migrated from Punjab to Tanzania when they were younger are structured accounts with a beginning, middle, and end that incorporate diversity of experiences. Mand (2006: 1058) and colleagues found that the narratives revealed:

> a gendered African space, which for men revolves around risk and adventure while for women Africa is experienced in the context of familial relations. Through elderly Sikh men and women's narratives about arrival in Tanzania we learn about the complex negotiations that occur based on gender and ethnic identity between and within families.

Gubrium (1990) observed metatheorizing by participants in support groups for caregivers of people with Alzheimer's disease in the United States. He believed that changes in participants' activities were evidence of personality adjustment to caregiving and success in overcoming obstacles to communicating thoughts and feelings. Obstacles to participants' reflective processes were overcome through use of poetry, and this provided access to the "heart" of the experience that the care equation, psychosocial stages, or scientific theorizing were less likely to provide (Gubrium 1990: 145–6). Gubrium (1990: 148) suggested that linkages between social gerontology and the humanities, for example providing opportunities for reflection through poetry, can offer opportunities for gerontologists to learn from ordinary reflection of older adults.

Radina, Hennon, and Gibbons (2008: 144) identified the importance of understanding process in order to learn about lived experiences of divorce. They emphasize the importance of "what the individual 'makes' of it; that is, the taken-for-granted world of one's family life and the language used to live within it and describe it to self and others" rather than divorce status. Nevertheless, "although people may share common localized cultures and thus family paradigms for making sense of their worlds as objective experiences, each person's marriage, divorce, and family worldview is distinctive and singular" (145–6).

Perspectives on narrative gerontology

Narrative gerontology is a phenomenological perspective that includes divergent views with one extreme arguing that narrative and experience precisely mirror each other and the diametrically opposed view that narrative provides very little resemblance to reality (Gubrium 2001: 19). Emphasizing focus rather than outcomes, Kenyon et al. (1999: 54) assert that narrative is study of lived experience or life world of an older adult. From the perspective of the individual, we are able to develop understanding of the social and interpersonal context that is made meaningful by the individual (Kenyon et al. 1999: 52).

Kenyon et al. suggest that the individual's personal context is especially important in the postmodern world where people may be separated from master narratives and no longer identify with these. They note that:

> We are only at the beginning of understanding the extent to which the story a person lives affects that person's quality of life and aging, biologically, psychologically, socially, and spiritually. We are only at the beginning of understanding the power of story-telling and storylistening in co-authoring each other's lives and experiencing the best that human life and aging has to offer.
>
> (Kenyon et al. 1999: 54)

According to Ewick and Silbey (1995), narrative analysis may reveal truths about the social world that may not be evident when more traditional methods of social science and legal scholarship are used. Narrative gerontology proposes that all aspects of the social world, including social identities and social action, are storied. Narrative is constitutive of that which it represents. In contrast, examination of lives, experiences, consciousness, or action outside of the narratives that constitute them is believed to deprive events and persons of meaning by distortion through abstraction and removal form their contexts.

Narrative analysis is also celebrated for overtly political reasons because narratives are considered by some scholars to have transformative or subversive potential. Narrative studies intend to give voice to the subject, and narrative scholarship can rewrite social life in ways that can be liberatory (Ewick and Silbey 1995). Narratives can acknowledge the legitimacy of diverse experiences and perspectives.

Metaphors in narrative gerontology

Kenyon et al. (1999) consider the term "narrative gerontology" to be a root metaphor, or heuristic. In this capacity, narrative gerontology gathers certain insights about aging and its study. They view the most important insight to be "explication of the implications of the 'life as story' metaphor for theory, research, and practice in the field of aging" (1999: 40–1) and describe four characteristics of the narrative gerontology root metaphor. The first characteristic is narrative gerontology's presupposition of an existential-ontological image of human beings as storytellers and storylisteners. Life stories are perceived to possess cognitive, affective, and volitional dimensions. Human beings are regarded to "be stories," thinking, perceiving, and acting on the basis of stories.

The second characteristic of the narrative gerontology root metaphor is that lives and lifestyles are made up of facticity. This is considered to include the "outside aspects of the stories we are, such as the social and structural dimensions of stories described in the next characteristic of the metaphor, as well as the story that we tell ourselves (and therefore are) at any moment in time" (Kenyon et al. 1999: 40). However, in contrast to facticity, stories also include inner aspects of possibility that inner aspects of a story and a life are subject to change and choice, new meaning, or "re-storying." Re-storying refers to people enhancing their sense of possibility by telling, reading, and retelling their life stories.

According to Kenyon et al. (1999), there are four interrelated dimensions in our lives as lifestories. The first is a structured story that includes aspects such as social policy and power relations. Structural constraints (part of facticity) can effectively silence voices, personal stories, voices, and the sense of possibility. The second is a sociocultural story or social meanings associated with aging and the life course. These include such things as professional-client and employer-worker relationships and cultural, ethnic, and gender stories. The third is an interpersonal dimension that includes intimate relationships such as those of confidants, families, and in which love is experienced. The fourth dimension pertains to the personal dimension of a lifestory itself. This dimension consists of the creation and discovery of meaning and coherence.

The fourth characteristic of the narrative gerontology root metaphor is the unique, idiosyncratic, and unknowable nature of the personal story. Kenyon et al. (1999: 41) suggest that the "moment of meaning for a person contains a distinctly inner existential-spiritual quality at the same time that meaning is created/discovered in a fundamentally paradoxical social and interpersonal context." Of course, people can and do communicate and learn a great deal about themselves and others, but narrative gerontology claims that we will never have the entire truth about life.

Implications of narrative gerontology for theories and research about aging

Kenyon et al. (1999: 42–3) have identified implications of a narrative gerontology for theories of aging. They suggest that other disciplines and gerontology generally have used narratives from a modern science perspective to access data considered subjective. In the modern science approach, "narratives are employed as a way to get at the most subjective aspects of a reality of aging that lies objectively behind the scenes and has its own rules." The method may guide the research problem rather than the problem guiding the research approach. In contrast, narrative gerontology as conceptualized by Kenyon et al. contributes the postmodern insight that:

> all knowledge is metaphorical, historical, and contextual...In other words, it is storied. Among other things, this means that all theories of aging are narratives; that is what is meant by the term *hermeneutic circle*...the hermeneutic circle constitutes the bottom line...As Carr (1986) notes, 'There is nothing below the narrative structure, as least nothing experienceable by us or comprehensible in experiential terms.'
>
> (Kenyon et al.1999: 66)

According to Kenyon et al. (1999: 42–3), this view suggests that theories of aging or formal intervention strategies as human activities:

> ...always contain a story with implicit and/or explicit meanings or ontological images of human nature, its development, and its teleology. This postmodern argument is in distinct contrast to the modern science claims that the facts will 'out' as long as one follows the scientific method and that there is both the possibility and necessity for objectivity in science. Rather, our argument here is that researchers and interveners bring their own stories (and values) to the professional situation, and those meanings and values are important components of what comes to count as valid knowledge of aging, as a good theory, as an appropriate intervention strategy, or as sound policy.

They suggest that in reality socially constructed theories and methods can guide the phenomenon to be investigated rather than the problem suggesting the appropriate study method, and this is not acceptable.

Approaching continuity theory from a narrative perspective, Kenyon and colleagues (1999: 46) use their perception of assumptions in continuity theory to speculate whether continuity theory is about:

> aging per se or whether is some cases it reflects a cohort, cultural, or period effect based on a widespread belief in a linear view of time that has created a 'bondage to the past'...There are significant differences in an understanding of aging based on, on the one hand, outer or clock time and, on the other hand, inner or story time.

Consistent with narrative gerontology, Kenyon et al. (1999: 46) point out that stories of older people involve a past dimension but are re-storied for present purposes:

> People ascribe present meaning to or express present metaphors of past events. In one sense the past exists only as it is remembered and created and re-created in the interaction with present and future experiences and with the meaning, interpretations, and metaphors ascribed to those experiences.... It would be interesting to look at the way in which people of different ages and cohorts 'story' and re-story time.

Kenyon et al. (1999: 51) suggest that, "The activity of recovering meaning consists of making the 'perceptual turn' to viewing a particular phenomenon 'as a story,' whether that phenomenon is a scientific theory or method or one's own life." This is called the re-storying moment, and examples of radical re-storying include experiences of some widows and victims of abuse, incest, and cancer that demonstrate the resiliency of the human spirit.

Kenyon et al. (1999: 44) recommend vantage points for development of theory and research:

1. Given the existential-ontological nature of narratives, it becomes important to investigate how theories are constructed in gerontology. For example, if there is no absolute reality, then we can ask whether knowledge of aging is, on the one hand, completely relative to a group and exclusively socially constructed or, on the other hand, an interpersonal and cultural co-authoring process based on a dialogue with many constituent epistemological variables.
2. A further research question concerns the elements of the story of theory construction in gerontology. The autobiographies of gerontological theorists could be analyzed to understand the contributions of different dimensions of their own lifestories to a better understanding of both aging and theories of aging.
3. We could inquire as to the nature of truth from a narrative gerontology perspective to distinguish appropriate from inappropriate theoretical stories to guide research and practice and thereby explicate the fundamental importance of the inside of aging to theorizing. A further related question is whether there is a moral imperative to knowledge of aging.
4. There may be some important education and training issues associated with theory construction in gerontology in terms of the range of conceptual frameworks to which students are exposed and which they are encouraged to explore....In gerontology it could be the case that the broader the exposure or the bigger the story, the better the theory, even though ultimately more specialized themes are adopted by gerontologists in their graduate work and professional life.

Research example: Narrative interpretation: "I'm on my way: the meaning of being oldest old, as narrated by people aged 95 and older"

In "I'm on My Way: The Meaning of Being Oldest Old, as Narrated by People Aged 95 and Older," Fischer et al. (2007) present a phenomenological hermeneutic analysis of interviews with 12 people between the ages of 95 and 103. The participants were the oldest respondents in the Umea 85+ Study in Northern Sweden focusing on health and life outlook. Their analysis implemented a method that was used previously by Lindseth and Norberg (2004), Rasmussen et al. (1995), Soderberg et al. (1999), and Sundin et al. (2002). This required a dialectical process "between approaching the text as a whole and approaching its parts, between understanding and explaining, and between focusing on what the text says and on what it points to" (Fischer et al. 2007: 7). The interpretive process was accomplished in three steps.

The first step involved reading the interview content to develop naïve understanding. This provided a broad understanding regarding what it meant to the respondents to be among the oldest old. The second step was structural analysis "which was done to explain and give depth to the interpretation, and to validate or invalidate the naïve understanding, involved a process in which each interview text was divided into meaning units, which could be anything in length from a phrase to several paragraphs. Next, the meaning units were condensed while still preserving the core. After this process, subthemes and themes were developed." Third, knowledge from naïve understanding, structural analysis, and researchers' preunderstanding and review of relevant literature was used to formulate a comprehensive understanding of meanings of being oldest old (Fischer et al. 2007: 7–8):

> Reading the interview texts for naïve understanding provided the following information: The text revealed an image of being at the end of one's life, at the end of a lived continuum. This is described as not being able to get around as before, and being in a limiting body. Despite the aches and pains and hindrances, there are possibilities to have time to reflect on life and to reminisce. The pondering can lead to an insight shaped by thankfulness for having had a good life, and absence of bitterness. Finally, the texts revealed consciousness of the inevitable fact that death is short at hand. Though enhancing death as a natural order in life and a move toward something else, often described as heaven or a 'better land,' the texts revealed anxiety about what was going to happen at the time preceding death.
>
> (Fischer et al. 2007: 8)

Structural analysis revealed two themes, being in stillness and movement, and four subthemes. Stillness relates to stiffness of the body and the soul's peacefulness, and movement refers to inner movement of memories and thoughts. Being in stillness was described as:

> Being oldest old means to be in one's limited body, and not being able to move as before. The body is still, immovable, tired, fatigued, and feels heavy to use. It is not as easy as before to get well after being in bad shape. 'The body stops you'; 'you can't bend down.' The aches and pains in both the legs and the spine are a hindrance. 'You can feel that you are getting worse and feeble.' The sight and hearing have declined and make it impossible to enjoy what one used to enjoy doing. 'Sometimes it feels very exhausting, I feel I have no energy.'
>
> The changes in the body mean having to stop doing certain things. The oldest old person is in need of help and assistance in performance of many tasks. 'I've stopped getting up on the ladder,' as one of the respondents revealed. The weariness is obvious. Even if the body is

not all immovable there are concerns about how to keep fit, how to maintain the mobility in the joints to prevent stiffness or do exercise every day in spite of age, 'I think I live just by having stood up in the morning.'

The stillness these oldest old persons are in is also a stillness of the older person, the quietness of the soul. The texts revealed the meaning of being in one's thoughts and dreams, by oneself. It means to just sit and wait and not do anything, 'so I can sit and just let the thoughts wander' and 'I can sit here for a couple of hours...almost asleep.' Some of the interviewees said that it is wonderful to be able to sleep. 'I get lost far away in my thoughts, I float around, it is like being in another world. When one is old one does not think so much what to do...one rests in a way – vegetates, I used to say.'

Friends and family die. 'Few are left in one's own age group.' – you are left alone. Loneliness is a problem if you are left alone, abandoned. However, being by yourself is also positive. 'One needs a little calmness and peaceful moments too...yes, really pray thoroughly, now when I'm alone I can open my heart....and it feels good to be alone.' One interviewee said, 'I do feel peace and serenity, yes I do.'

(Fischer et al. 2007: 9)

The other dominant theme is movement, and this included subthemes or reminiscence and engagement in inner dialogue, being at the end of life and contemplating the future, moving to a "better land," and being confident that they would be taken care of but experiencing anxiety about the process of dying rather than death itself.

Being oldest old, being in a body that is still, can also bring inner movement, sometimes even agility. This can happen when old people lie down to rest or sleep, since they enter into the memories that float back from the past: 'It is just like in the movies. You lie awake in the night and then...[the memories] roll up again.' You remember everything, both good and bad. The texts revealed that the interviewees reminisced much, and that reminiscing is a powerful experience that is very strong and intense and touches and moves beyond time and space. 'Yes, very often it is that I'm back in the world of my youth and childhood. I'm back in all the old; I live with it so strongly that it feels like I'm there.... I shut out the present...live back...you relive your youth and childhood like that.' Some interviewees said that during such intense reminiscing, it was possible to meet, and feel the nearness of, their deceased spouses – 'She is with me, she is here.' Some of them said this challenged their thinking.

There can also be more to remember than was expected and this awakens thoughts that are swift and movable. 'When one is still, and lies down, the thoughts come' – 'Yes, you should understand, the thoughts move along very long and winding roads....I think of all different things.' The thinking and pondering take place as an inner dialogue. People go through and think of what they have done and left undone. 'I explain to myself why I think like this...and then I have to grasp.' This process can lead to reevaluating life into an insight shaped by thankfulness and absence of bitterness, as well as reconciliation with one's life. 'I used to say like this that I have become richer inside. You understand quite new values...a richness.' Thinking and pondering can be arduous and the interviewees talked about a conscious effort to hold onto the good memories and force oneself to forget and hold other thoughts back. 'There is so much here inside that I can't put it into words.' However, 'now is the time to think,' as one oldest old person said. This thinking and pondering also concerns the changes in society. So much had changed within the interviewees' lifetimes. They felt that now was a new era, and that there were so many new things that they would not experience any more. Life was at its end.

(Fischer et al. 2007: 10, 11)

Diversity and ways of aging

Jaber Gubrium (2003) and many other proponents of his phenomenological approach to study of aging have addressed diversity of experiences in aging. They have identified aspects of identities of older people that are shaped by social, cultural, and material contexts and expressed in persistence, adaptation, and change. Examples of narratives and their interpretations reflecting diversity of aging experiences include narratives reflecting identity careers of older gay men and lesbians and narratives of forgiveness in old age.

Research example: identity careers of older gay men and lesbians

Dana Rosenfeld (2003: 161) conducted open-ended, in-depth interviews with 50 ethnically and socioeconomically diverse gay men and lesbians in the Los Angeles area when they were between the ages of 64 and 89 in 1995. She identified the narrative paths of participants who developed their identities during the separate historical periods before and after the gay liberation movement in the United States during the 1960s and 1970s. Societal perceptions and responses to homosexuality when the participants were middle aged and younger considered this to be a medical, moral, and legal aberration. Their recollections of sexual experiences and identity issues were influenced by experiences in their earlier lives when homosexuality was "exclusively constructed as a shameful stigma and a new period in which being gay was increasingly viewed as a positive identity." A central theme of the interviews was that their identities were formed when there was tremendous social change, and their "identity careers" in life narrative paths into later adulthood continued to be shaped by these events.

According to Rosenfeld (2003: 161), the interviews document identity careers that "reflect ways of aging mediated by changing understandings of what might be considered the proper interpretation and enactment of sexual desire." She suggests that this is consistent with C. Wright Mills's (1959) argument that biographical narratives are shaped in form and content by ideas and values of specific historical times in which they exist. Rosenfeld (2003: 165) suggests in their earlier years:

> the stigmatizing discourse of the times provoked the challenge of making the self intelligible and, at the same time, preserving its value in the face of a devalued identity. Subjects described feeling caught between a need to understand and pursue their desires on the one hand and to avoid the negative implications of a stigmatized identity on the other. Recognizing and fulfilling sexual desires served to discredit them, making them subject to ridicule and rejection.

Earlier in life, most of the older adults in Rosenfeld's study had identified as homosexual in a manner consistent with the stigmatized formulation and had passed as heterosexual in public, but some did not identify themselves as gay or lesbian despite their attraction to members of the same gender. Later they began to identify as homosexual when a new homosexual identity became available. They tried to understand their differences:

> Most subjects spoke of searching for accounts of these differences in textual and cultural representations and in others' remarks. For example, Rodney, aged 81, wrote to the editor and publisher of a homoerotic 'muscle' magazine for advice to 'determine where I stood in life.' Jeannine, age 66, and her female lover searched the dictionary for female versions of the word 'faggot.' Others described pondering their interactions and characterizations to uncover the nature and consequences of their desires. Without exception, the accounts formulated same-sex desires as a pathological yet curable condition.

This discourse 'explained' subjects' experiences to them in stigmatizing terms, and thus supplied a much-needed identity category....

The stigmatizing discourse of the times provoked the challenge of making the self intelligible and, at the same time, preserving its value in the face of a devalued identity. Subjects described feeling caught between a need to understand and pursue their desires on the one hand and to avoid the negative implications of a stigmatized identity on the other. Recognizing and fulfilling sexual desires served to discredit them, making them subject to ridicule and rejection.

(Rosenfeld 2003: 164–5)

When they were younger, many respondents had distanced themselves from interpreting their desires in terms of a stigmatized homosexual identity and the consequences of acting on them by making their same-sex desire less important than interests, needs, and obligations perceived to provide greater rewards. Others coped by pursuing heterosexual relationships and developing a heterosexual identity. Some respondents who had not known how to interpret their homosexual desires described their initial sexual or erotic contacts as providing insight into their desires and how to fulfill them. Meeting and associating with other homosexuals also assisted interpretation of their desires and reduced feelings of isolation. Many developed emotional needs that only same-sex erotic or romantic relationships could satisfy. The social movements in the 1970s provided a broad social context for forming new relationships and a new symbolic framework for understanding themselves.

Respondents shared their views about being old and lesbian or gay. Some considered homosexuality to be relevant to old age while others did not:

William, age 76, said 'Some people, both gay and heterosexual, age gracefully and some don't. And I don't know that being gay has anything specifically to do with it.'... For Kate, aged 76, the circumstances under which people age center on social support, which she felt is independent of sexuality. As she explained, the isolation of the older person depends upon whether they ever married or had children, what kind of families they have. A straight woman who never married, if she has a loving niece, you know, great. If she doesn't, too damned bad. I think it's a matter of old age per se and the kind of friends and the kind of family you have. It's a question of you're single, you damned well better have a support system and/or some sort of family. You know most people that are my age and single do have nieces and nephews, you see. Having been a single child I don't have that. I think that cuts across the whole society in terms of old age.

(Rosenfeld 2003: 178–9)

Other respondents regretted that they did not have the support system provided by the traditional family, but several said that absence of conventional family relations provided freedom from some constraints and concerns: For 68-year-old Jan, childlessness is said to free older homosexuals from children's constant reminder of their relatively advanced age, resulting in subjective feelings of youthfulness.

> I don't think of myself as old, elderly or even aging. And I think if I were in the regular mode – a husband and kids, grandchildren – I'd have grandchildren at this point, and a constant reminder from all these years that have crept up and having all these generations younger than myself would tend to feel much older I think than perhaps I do now. [Heterosexuals] usually do age faster.
>
> (Rosenfeld 2003: 177)

Luke, age 69, considered older heterosexuals to be vulnerable to the wishes of members of their traditional families and at risk for institutionalization by their children:

> Their sons and daughters take them and make them lonelier by putting them in convalescent homes and getting rid of them. When you're gay, no one can do that to you, you have to do it to yourself. So you go on by yourself until you don't have any more strength to go on. And that's why I'm 68 and I still feel like I'm 55.
>
> (Rosenfeld 2003: 178)

Biographies of future cohorts of lesbian and gay older adults will be influenced by life in new historical eras in which there are significant social changes. Rosenfeld (2003: 179) suggests that discussion about the shape of lesbian and gay families, as well as newly developed same-sex partner benefits that allow additional degrees of financial and legal commitment, have important implications for security in old age. In contrast to the 1950s, gay men and lesbians can be open about their sexual orientation at their place of employment and not be legally dismissed because of their sexual orientation. Gay voting blocs and lobbying efforts will provide opportunities for development of diverse public identities. Rosenfeld (2003: 179) continues:

> Accompanying this is the explosion of venues for the discussion and contesting of homosexual identity in the mass media, which suggests that future cohorts of older gay men and lesbians will have devoted a shorter period of their lives to identify issues surrounding their sexuality. It is doubtful that today's teenagers experiencing same-sex desires will spend as much time plowing through a discourse of difference

to interpret their desires. Indeed, the now classic coming out story may become less dramatic and less painful than it has been, one which seems to have been a narrative watershed for the older subjects of the generation under consideration.

Research example: narratives of forgiveness in old age

Helen K. Black (2003) found differences in experiences of forgiveness in old age as she listened to the stories of 40 African American and Caucasian men and women age 70 and over. While it is commonly assumed that forgiveness of self or others should occur in old age, Black found that forgiveness is not a simple developmental imperative (Black 2001, 2003) but is embedded in an elder's past, present, and anticipated future (Black 2003). The extent to which the perceived wrong continued to affect the elder and whether the perpetrator remained in the elder's life was found by Black to affect whether or not forgiveness occurred. Furthermore, the elder's "personal past, cohort history, and the cultural, ethnic, racial, and religious traditions" mediate the individual's need to resolve wrongs (Snowden 2001, in Black 2003: 13). Decisions by older people to forgive or withhold forgiveness can also be affected by the concrete event or incident in question (Calhoun 1992) and the life circumstances of the older adult (Black and Rubinstein 2000). Black presents narratives of Mr. Marks and Miss Mel as examples of variations in forgiveness in later adulthood.

"Mr. Marks"

In "Narratives of Forgiveness in Old Age" (2003), Black describes Mr. Marks, a 72-year-old semi-retired married man living near Philadelphia with his wife of 51 years. He recounted that he grew up in Philadelphia, continued to live there after his marriage, and joined his father's retail business after working in his father-in-law's upholstery business.

Black (2003: 15) suggests that since Mr. Marks began his narrative by talking about work, this indicates "the salience of work in his life as well as the belief that work is a legacy both to inherit and bequeath."

Mr. Marks and his wife had three sons, and Mr. Marks described Jeb, the youngest, as different from his brothers. Education was stressed in the home, and the oldest sons became a doctor and a biomedical researcher, while Jeb struggled academically. However, Jeb attended college and married a classmate, and their son was born a year after their graduation.

When Jeb had difficulty finding employment after graduation, he asked to join the family business, and Mr. Marks was delighted that the business would be owned and managed by a third generation. However, Jeb became ill with cancer and lived only 10 months after his diagnosis. While talking about Jeb's illness, Mr. Marx "displays little emotion... but clips his words, breaks off at mid-sentence, looks away from the interviewer, and glances around the bright kitchen" (Black 2003: 16).

Mr. Marks never mentioned Jeb's wife by name during the interview, but in his story about forgiveness she is the person who he could not forgive for what happened after Jeb's death. Mr. and Mrs. Marks had paid the entire cost of a life insurance policy for Jeb that was worth $800,000, and although they had not intended for the money to come to them, Jeb's wife was suing them for the money. His daughter-in-law was also considered unforgivable because she prevented him from access to his memories of Jeb and to Jeb's son, Tim. He was denied the sense of generativity and legacy that was important to him. She kept their grandson, Tim, away from them, and they had to hide themselves when trying to glimpse him. According to Black, the fact that his daughter-in-law consciously and willfully made decisions that are hurtful to Mr. Marks and wife and his inability to understand her motivation have contributed to his inability to forgive her actions. She remains a presence in their lives due to ongoing lawsuits, and he sees no likelihood of repentance on her part or an end to his pain. Black notes that the comment "It eats at me" is frequently repeated in stories about forgiveness told by elders and that physical manifestations often accompany psychological responses. Mr. Marks had a painful ulcer; other respondents have described weight loss for which there is no diagnosed cause.

When he was asked to describe "other incidents, events, or stories about forgiveness" he discussed his work in the United States military as a warden in Nuremberg, Germany, at the end of World War II, guarding high-level Nazi officers tried for war crimes (Black 2003: 18). Black notes that the word forgiveness is not used in this narrative. She perceived that:

> lurking between the story's lines is a surprised and troubled wonder about his lack of conscious thought and feeling while at Nuremberg....
> [Later in life] Mr. Marks views the prisoners' genocide, [the prison psychologist's insight in a book written later based on conversations with the prisoners], and the significance of his role at Nuremberg with the vantage of time. He initially thought that the psychologist's job was 'boring.' Perhaps for Marks, to attempt to 'get into anyone's mind' seems a thankless and mostly unfulfilling task.... However,

agreeing with the psychologist's insight showed that he formed deep and lasting perceptions about the prisoners he guarded.

(Black 2003: 18, 19)

Mr. Marks believes that it is more difficult to forgive as one becomes older because life becomes more difficult in old age. His personal attitude is that as a Jewish man he does not want to forgive, and Black suggests that Mr. Marks's statements about his personal perspectives as a Jewish man provide insight for understanding his attitudes about forgiveness. Black demonstrates that phenomenological study of life experiences contributing to Mr. Marks's attitudes about forgiveness support understanding of his inability to forgive his daughter-in-law. She concludes that age has not altered his view of himself or his beliefs about who should be forgiven or why. According to Black (2003: 21–2), Mr. Marks's description of forgiveness is rooted in "concrete and profound experiences of his life and in his personal inability to 'see' or 'picture' a reason or resolution for these realities. His definition of forgiveness reiterates his continuing questions about the horrors and injustices of life: 'Let bygones be bygones. But don't forgive. I mean, how can you? You can't obliterate your memories. They're real. How do you forgive?'"

"Miss Mel"

Black (2003) also describes the narrative of forgiveness of Miss Mel, an 80-year-old African American woman who lives in a home that she owns in Philadelphia. She has difficulty walking and therefore leaves her door unlocked for visitors including her nephew, niece, social workers, and delivery staff for home-delivered meals. Her neighbors look out for her safety. Miss Mel worked in a hotel and then received training for nursing work and did this work until retirement. Responding to interviewer prompts for more information about her childhood and young adulthood, Miss Mel said that her early life in the Southern United States included some bad times that she remembers, but these had become good memories because they were a reminder of how far she had come. She said that she keeps these experiences to herself because God has given her peace of mind. According to Black, Miss Mel was reluctant to dwell on unpleasant experiences in her past and transformed negative situations by considering them to be useful or instructional. Bad times could become good memories if they were useful learning experiences. They were considered especially valuable if they were overcome.

Miss Mel had two sons with her first husband, and her two marriages ended in divorce. Her oldest son is incarcerated, and her youngest son is studying for the ministry. Referring to her son's incarceration, Miss Mel says:

> Justice is not equal. Don't you see the scale of justice? It's always uneven. And see the one that's in prison is dark like I am; it would all be different if he wasn't so black. Because my younger son was a drug addict and now he's studying for the ministry. He could get a job anywhere. He's accepted anywhere. But not the dark one.
>
> (Black 2003: 29)

Black's (2003: 29–30) interpretation of this segment of Miss Mel's story is:

> She is aware of the cultural realities that make social equality improbable if not impossible for her older son. However, she makes it clear that there is a higher justice in which she places her trust.... Despite feeling that his very 'blackness' makes him appear guilty to a jury, she explains that she is concerned but not worried about the outcome of the parole board's decision: 'I'm 80 years old now and I've come a long, long way through a lot of trials. I seen a lot. With God – all things, not some – all things are possible. And this is what I depend on'...because her strength and her wealth are spiritual and she has joyfully shared her largesse with others, she believes that she will be rewarded with an affirmative answer to her prayer about her son's release.

Discussing her need to forgive her first husband's infidelity and long-term relationship with Belle, a member of their church, Miss Mel described her need to forgive herself, perhaps for a vengeful altercation with Belle, and also forgive her husband and his lover. She described lifting herself out of hatred:

> I told Belle..., 'Go ahead. We'll just have my husband together.' [Pause] That was a terrible, terrible thing! I was letting myself down to no esteem whatsoever. Because I knew it was wrong for me to share my husband and take abuse from an outside woman. I was letting her do it to me. I sat there and I said, 'Mel, you're a nothing.' When you can analyze yourself this way, then you realize that you've got to come up. You cannot stay down below the line of self-respect. I had lost that. 'Mel, you're a nothing.'
>
> (Black 2003: 31)

Miss Mel targeted Belle with much greater blame than her husband for the extramarital relationship because she regarded her husband as weak and believed that it was Belle who could have stopped the relationship.

Nevertheless, Miss Mel's path to self-respect included forgiveness of Belle:

> Well, I went back to the church and I became the president of the church club. And I just trusted in God. I appointed Belle as the secretary. It took one year and then I woke up one morning and I didn't hate nobody. And I called her and I said, 'Belle, how you feeling this morning?' She said 'All right.' I said, "I want to tell you something. I don't hate you no more. I love you.' She said, 'I never did hate you.' I said, 'Well, I sure hated you.'
>
> (Black 2003: 31–2)

According to Black (2003: 32–3):

> She links forgiveness to acknowledging her hatred and apologizing to the 'hated' party even if that person is the perpetrator of the wrong. Ultimately, she connects forgiveness with self-esteem. In fact, as she encouraged church members to be kind to Belle, she believes she was lifted to a 'sacred place' where she could 'forgive anybody anything'...Miss Mel believes that her capacity to forgive enlarged with age....
>
> Miss Mel's way of forgiving seems, to the interviewer, as complex and circuitous as her self-described way of aging, and indeed, her way of living. Her way of forgiving is embedded in cultural and racial traditions concerning appropriate behaviors for men and women, and in the belief that personal spirituality is transformative.

Summary

The foundation of social phenomenology that provides the basis for development of phenomenological gerontology is the work of European philosophers Edmund Husserl, Martin Heidegger, Gabriel Marcel, Simone de Beauvoir, Maurice Merleau-Ponty, and Jean-Paul Sartre. Phenomenology has continued to be influenced by Husserl's belief that the phenomenologist suspends belief in the existence of the outer world, things within it, and validity of statements about the world for his analytical purpose, suspending belief in its existence, in order to refrain intentionally and systematically from all judgments related to the existence of the outer world.

Albert Schutz made important theoretical contributions to the development of phenomenology, including his emphasis on the social construction of reality, and brought phenomenology to the United States during the 1930s. Schutz connected

Husserl's conceptualization of phenomenology to Max Weber's conceptualization of the ideal type, and this contributed to Schutz's formulation of phenomenological analysis. Processes that Schutz considered to be first-order typifications in which a shared social world is constructed as people bring together enduring and typical experiences create the basis of second-order typifications that are rational intellectual models of the social world based on the first-order typifications.

In phenomenological gerontology, it is theorized that knowledge that is useful for developing understanding is available in narratives provided by older people. Phenomenological approaches in aging studies contrast sharply with the biomedical model that focuses primarily on bodily failures. Sociologists Jaber Gubrium and James Holstein's approaches to theory development and research are based on the idea that understanding can be achieved through exploration of ordinary ways that older people experience daily life, manage successes and failures, and construct their past and future in relation to the present. Supportive of a focus on diversity of experiences, Gubrium and Holstein believe that individual meanings of old age are connected to continuing aspects of a person's biography that make it possible for affirmative construction of later life. This is exemplified in Rosenfeld's descriptions of identity development of older gay men and lesbian women and Black's descriptions of narratives of forgiveness in old age.

The reality that older adults engage in metatheorizing as reflection on their activities is a key aspect of phenomenological gerontology. Narrative construction is viewed as dynamic so that interpretation of one's own experiences can change over time through individuals' ordinary theorizing. Narrative gerontology is an approach to understanding later adulthood from a phenomenological perspective and is theorized to have a root metaphor with four characteristics: presupposition of an existential-ontological image of human beings as storytellers and storylisteners who are stories; lives and lifestyles are made up of facticity but re-storying can also occur; interrelated dimensions consisting of a structured story, a sociocultural story, interpersonal dimensions, and personal dimensions; and a personal story is to some extent idiosyncratic, unique, and unknowable. Narrative gerontology suggests research topics that include the following: how theories are constructed in gerontology; the elements of the story of theory construction in gerontology, including the influence of lifestories of theorists; the nature of truth from a narrative gerontology perspective in order to distinguish inappropriate from appropriate theoretical stories to guide research and practice; and education and training issues regarding the range of conceptual frameworks associated with theory construction in gerontology.

Fischer, Norbeg, and Lundman's phenomenological hermeneutic analysis of interviews with people between the ages of 95 and 103 in Northern Sweden provides an example of narrative analysis as a dialectical process in which interpretation was accomplished in three steps. Their analysis involved reading the interview content to develop naïve understanding providing a sense of the whole about the meaning to the respondents of being among the oldest old. This was followed by structural analysis to explain and provide depth to the interpretation and validate or invalidate the naïve understanding. Meaning units were condensed while the core was preserved, and themes and subthemes developed. Lastly, researchers' preunderstanding and review of relevant literature, knowledge from naïve understanding, and structural analysis was used to formulate understanding of meanings of being oldest old.

4 Critical gerontology

Key concepts

1. Critical gerontology is influenced primarily by the work of first generation Frankfurt School theorists Theodor Adorno and Max Horkheimer, second generation theorist Jurgen Habermas, and by Michel Foucault's post-structuralist theoretical perspectives.
2. Critical perspectives in contemporary social gerontology are driven by concern and include political economy of aging, feminist gerontology, humanistic gerontology, theories of diversity, and specific social constructionist approaches.
3. Influenced primarily by the Frankfurt School of critical theory and Foucault's post-structuralism, critical gerontology focuses on criticism of the process of power.
4. Postmodern trends that resulted in demand for a critical approach to gerontology included concern about the disease model of aging, the generational equity debate, and the mood of cost containment.
5. The political economy perspective proposes that economic dependency is not primarily the result of chronological age but also results from relationships between age and labor market and age and the welfare state that are socially constructed.
6. In the political economy perspective, characteristics such as gender, race, and class are considered pivotal variables in aging because they predetermine a person's location in the social order.
7. Wang's critical analysis of the "American seniors' movement" and alternative forms of resistance by older Chinese women and others is informed by Foucault's model of power/subject/resistance.
8. Maggie Kuhn and the Gray Panthers worked to change structures of domination through approaches that were consistent with a critical approach intended to define and achieve a meaningful context for later adulthood.

Introduction

Chapter 4 provides an introduction to critical theory and description of critical gerontology, including British sociologist Alan Walker's critical analysis of old age and development of the welfare state. The chapter also includes Frank T.Y. Wang's critical analysis of development of the "American seniors' movement" in the United States and his critical analysis of suicide among older Chinese women as an alternative form of resistance. Both are analyzed in terms of critical concepts in Michel Foucault's theories. The chapter concludes with discussion of the activism of the Gray Panthers organization in the United States and its founder, Maggie Kuhn, from the perspective of critical theory.

Foundations of critical theory

Critical theory in gerontology is influenced primarily by the work of first genera-tion Frankfurt School theorists Theodor Adorno and Max Horkheimer, second generation theorist Jurgen Habermas, and by Michel Foucault's post-structuralist theoretical perspectives. Frankfurt School theorists differentiated between reason that they considered instrumental and reason considered enlightening and eman-cipating and strongly preferred the latter. They thought that instrumental reason unreflectively supports effective means for any accepted purpose and was mani-fested in technocratic thinking that dominated industrialization and adminis-tration during the 1900s. In contrast, enlightening and emancipating reason was influenced by ideals of the French Revolution; justice, peace, and happiness were preferred for measuring human conditions (Landmann 1977: xi).

Frankfurt School theorists accused positivistic/empirical sociology of glorify-ing whatever exists and criticized positivistic sociology's acceptance of social facts as quasi-neutral. They believed that social facts should be explored within their context of structural interconnections reflecting the totality of society and its movement, and they were concerned about positivistic sociology's readiness to accept social facts in a value-free manner. They considered modern society's domination of nature unjustifiable and desired reconciliation with nature through nonexploitative technology (Landmann 1977: x–xi).

Foucault's initial development of his post-structuralist approach was strongly influenced by ideas of playwright Samuel Beckett and philosopher Friedrich Nietzsche. All three challenged the practice of modern understanding of truth and knowledge established by seventeenth-century French philosopher and math-ematician René Descartes. Descartes considered philosophy analogous to a tree with roots in metaphysics, the trunk as physics, and branches representing differ-ent sciences. Consistent with the tree metaphor, Descartes considered all knowl-edge to have an essential unity and viewed philosophy as raising a canopy of useful postulates for ordinary living. The practical sciences were viewed as fruits at the end of the branches, and he wrote that people should acquire knowl-edge that would enable them to master and possess nature. He compared meta-physics, which he considered the first philosophy, to a tree's roots, positing that development of knowledge must be from the bottom and based on first principles (Irving 1999).

Foucault was especially critical of Descartes's concepts of philosophical foundationalism (Descartes's famous "Method") and intuitional normativism. The premise of philosophical foundationalism is that all genuine knowledge is based on a foundation of an indisputable first truth, such as the starting point of Descartes's system of knowledge. According to Descartes, all knowledge pursuant to this principle is valid if correctly reasoned. Institutional normativism, Descartes's idea of empiricism, refers to the idea that objective truth already exists and is waiting to be found. In contrast to Descartes's view of modernity, Foucault considered empirical reality to be contingent and historical, a collection of stories that people tell rather than a universal truth. Foucault's critical perspective, with its emphasis on the importance of personal stories, validates consideration of diversity of perspectives of realities constructed from language and cultural codes within invented institutions. Culturally conditioned paradigms provide diverse meanings to individuals' lives (Irving 1999: 32).

According to Prado (1995: 20):

> Foucault's denial that the historical accounts we give of disciplinary knowledge do or could capture objective progress is fundamental to his genealogical analysis. There is no story-independent progress that history discerns and describes because history records sequences of occurrences that power-relations determine to be significant events. This denial of an independent subject matter for history, a subject matter that historians might or might not correctly trace and record, perplexes many, often forcing them to adopt dubious interpretations of Foucault's genealogical work to make it more manageable and to mold it to their own expectations.

Critical gerontology

Concern was identified by Max Horkheimer, a Frankfurt School theorist, as arising from enlightened cognition through which the person becomes opposed to affirmative traditional theories (Putney et al. 2005: 94). Critical perspectives in contemporary social gerontology are driven by concern and include political economy of aging, feminist gerontology, humanistic gerontology, theories of diversity, and specific social constructionist approaches. Influenced primarily by the Frankfurt School of critical theory and Foucault's post-structuralism, critical gerontology focuses on criticism of the process of power (Putney et al. 2005: 94).

Moody (1993: xvii-xviii) identified postmodern trends in public discourse in the United States in the late twentieth century that resulted in demand for a critical approach to gerontology. These include biomedicalization of gerontology, the generational equity debate, the mood of cost containment, and nostalgia for positive images of old age amid awareness that there is more to aging than is reflected in the disease model of aging (Estes and Binney 1991). Structural components in critical gerontology include criticism of positivist knowledge and focus on strengths and diversity of old age (Bengtson et al. 1997).

Jecker (1993: 275) suggested that critical theory:

> invites and makes room for other perspectives by (1) questioning: turning criticism reflexively on oneself and one's traditions, theories, concepts, and methods; (2) enlarging: stretching traditional categories of thought to create an opening for change; and (3) unifying: revealing the extent to which apparently discordant ideas are interconnected.

The two patterns of study in critical gerontology have been: (1) humanistic dimensions of aging and (2) structural components of aging (Putney et al. 2005). Addressing the humanistic perspective, Moody (1993) differentiated critical gerontology from pragmatic liberalism, suggesting that pragmatic liberalism has been congenial to mainstream gerontology in the United States. In comparison to gerontology influenced by pragmatic liberalism, critical gerontology questions the idea that "interest group politics and value-free science promote well-being and progress for all" and that "interest-group politics and the market serve to reinforce a version of American pluralism that conceals systematic structures of domination and oppression" (Moody 1993: xv–xvi).

According to Fahey and Holstein (1993: 242), post-Enlightenment rational approaches to understanding have deterred gerontological researchers from probing normative and existential questions that could result in a new cultural vision for later adulthood. They recommended asking questions, including value questions, that are different from those permitted by dominant research methodologies; exploration in fields in addition to sociology and psychology; deductive and inductive analysis; and viewing older people as more than recipients of services. Consistent with a structural approach, the "explicit search for and defining of a meaningful context for this life stage – on the personal, societal, and species level – can be an important step in guiding individual aging, grounding public and private institutional and policy responses, and penetrating the resistant ageism that harms people of all ages" (Fahey and Holstein 1993: 255). Luborsky and Sankar (1993) suggested that the critical theory framework in gerontology needed to be extended to increase awareness within the field of gerontology and broaden the knowledge base pertaining to variables such as health, illness, ethnicity, family, self, and diversity in subgroup definitions of variables.

Substantial focus in critical gerontology has been devoted to issues pertaining to retirement policies. Atchley (1993) has proposed a challenge by critical gerontology of goals and beliefs forming the basis of retirement as a developing social institution. He suggested that Moody's (1988) meta-theoretical framework identifying critical theory, interpretive theory in hermeneutics, and analytical scientific theories can provide the foundation for critical analysis of assumptions pertaining to retirement. Atchley suggested that retirement was created to achieve social aims and is based on assumptions that the labor force must be reduced because production of necessary goods and services requires only a small proportion of adults able to do the work due to technological advances. Furthermore, retirement as a social institution assumes that people lose their value as workers as they become older, and a third assumption is that older adults leaving the labor market need retirement pensions since unemployment is socially disruptive.

According to Atchley, all of these assumptions can be challenged. Critical theorists can question the necessity for extensive automation that constrains and alienates workers. Likewise, the Taylorist perspective "that only the most desirable workers should be employed by industry" and the assumption that society does not need to find employment for everyone who wants to work can be questioned since there are prejudiced assumptions, including ageism, that limit the pool of people considered for employment (Atchley 1993: 6). Atchley (1993: 7) believes that the objective of

a critical gerontology of the institution of retirement, with its retirement rules, incentives, disincentives, and pension policies, is to expose further the deeper motives behind the institutions and to expose the patterns of domination contained within them. Once this has been accomplished, directions for emancipatory change can be identified and criticism can be focused on how such changes could be implemented.

Atchley (1993: 8) addresses retirement as a distributional issue because of its implications for distribution of jobs, income, and retirement opportunities. He notes (1993: 8):

The notion of organizing the economic life course into preparation, employment, and retirement has existed at least since the time of Plato, but the formal insertion of this life course into laws and rules morally justified the linkage between employment and retirement, especially in terms of social insurance retirement provisions. This linkage of employment and retirement also preserves into retirement the dominant system of status inequality. From this perspective, retirement is a major vehicle for achieving social integration among those who have been employed. But from the point of view of those who have had sporadic or nonexistent access to good jobs, access to retirement is limited.

Availability of retirement benefits varies substantially, and there is a bias in the U.S. toward long-term participants in the work force receiving the best retirement benefits (Atchley 1993).

In addition to addressing the reality that the prevailing pattern of economic and social domination in the U.S. constrains the ability of many workers to experience self-directed economic and social freedom in retirement, Atchley recommends that critical theorists explore the efficacy and availability of liberal educational opportunities for retirees that could support development of an emancipatory life stage. He also recommends exploration of opportunities for roles for retirees in criticism expressed through political and social organizations and attention by critical theorists to development of approaches to minimize coercive employment practices experienced by older adults (Atchley 1993).

Political economy perspective in critical gerontology

A new critical paradigm in social gerontology began to develop in the late 1970s in France, Great Britain, and the United States, and scholars who met at the World Congress of Sociology in Uppsala, Sweden, in 1978 produced elements of a new paradigm in 1979 and 1980. This paradigm was initially referred to as social construction of aging or structured dependency, subsequently called the political economy of aging, and finally critical gerontology. Early work in political economy of aging was developed primarily in response to functionalist theories suggesting that there were aspects of aging experiences, such as poverty, that were natural and inevitable in advanced industrial societies. The political economy response was that economic dependency is not primarily the result of chronological age but results from "socially constructed relationships between, principally, age and labor market and age and the welfare state" (Walker 2006: 60).

The political economy paradigm builds upon the Frankfurt theorists' view that scientific and political constructs recreate wider socio-historical environments (Luborsky and Sankar 1993). The broad implications of economic life for older people and for society's treatment of older adults are emphasized in the interdisciplinary and sociohistorical political economy perspective on aging and old age (Estes 1991). Sociohistorical, political, and economic factors influence perceptions of a group, including perceptions of older adults as a problem group (Estes 1991). In the political economy approach, two paths are followed. First, critical gerontology is considered an alternative to the instrumental orientation of academic gerontology and, secondly, interaction of political, socioeconomic, and other factors that shape and determine aging experiences are addressed (Ovrebo and Minkler 1993: 289).

In this perspective, characteristics such as gender, race, and class are considered pivotal variables in aging because they predetermine a person's location in the social order (Estes 1991; Ovrebo and Minkler 1993). According to British sociologist Alan Walker (2006: 60):

> This analysis had the effect of diverting the gerontological gaze away from the problems of old age and individual judgment to features of the aging process, towards structural constraints and sources of inclusion or exclusion such as pension policies, retirement policies, age discrimination, and so on. It emphasized structural inequalities between different groups of older people and focused on two key, but then neglected, aspects of the aging process: cumulative life-course advantages and disadvantages between different groups and the consequences of economic dependency on the state. ... It was seen by the scientific community as a radical departure and has provided the basis of an enormous flow of research in this field.

Alan Walker's critical perspective on old age and development of the welfare state

Walker emphasizes the relationship between old age and the welfare state in order to explain risk-society analysis and to counterbalance the narratives of biomedical and biological perspectives on aging and the emphasis on old age lifestyle and consumerism. He notes that there are strong historical connections between development of the welfare state and older adults. In European countries, by the early 1900s there was collective acknowledgement of old age as a risk status, and risk and definition of old age became institutionalized with the beginning of the postwar welfare state. However, the relationship between old age and the welfare state has varied, and Walker (2006: 61) asserts that "It is when we examine its dynamics that we can see the critical role of social policies and social institutions in structuring and restructuring the life course and the meaning of old age. Economic dependency and social exclusion have been socially constructed primarily by institutions such as the labor market and the welfare state."

Walker (2006: 62–3) has identified five consequences of institutionalization of age-related retirement in European countries from the 1940s to early 1970s and associated identification of old age as a social problem:

In the first place, the economic dependency of older people on the state was enlarged substantially. One hundred years ago in the United Kingdom, two-thirds of the male population age 65 and over were economically active (in employment or seeking it); today it is only 7%. Older people are not helpless pawns in this social definition of old age. On the contrary, individually and collectively, workers called for retirement and public pensions. But the creation of a fixed-age barrier in European pension systems led to widespread economic exclusion…in the second half of the twentieth century, large numbers of older workers opted for retirement before the fixed-age barrier, a choice that has become more widely available as pensions have risen in value.

Second, age-barrier retirement has been the main wellspring of age discrimination in employment, social security, and in wider social relations (Blytheway, 1995; McEwan, 1990…

Third, as a corollary to retirement, it has been accepted that the income needs of older people are lower than those of the 'economically active.'…

Fourth, age-barrier retirement and these foregoing factors have encouraged the view that older people are not just a social problem but an economic burden as well…

Fifth, with regard to health and social services policy and practice, it was this first phase that saw the major expansion of these services and their professionalization. Since policy makers had come to regard older people as largely dependent and passive objects, it is not surprising that the professional and institutional structures of the health and social services also tended to reflect this view...Thus the expansion of health and social services in this period was a two-sided coin: it enhanced the welfare of older people, but it was delivered in ways that reinforced their social and physical dependency and powerlessness.

Walker (2006: 63) describes the following phase, occurring from the beginning of fiscal crises in the mid-1970s to the late 1980s, as a transitional period, which he characterizes as "old age as a solution to one economic problem and the cause of another." During this period the social meaning of aging was reconstructed along two dimensions. Male economic activity in later life declined massively in all industrial countries except for Sweden and Japan, primarily among males age 60 and over, but declines also occurred among males between the ages of 55 and 59, and there appears to have been a similar decline among women. In Europe, this decline appears to have resulted from reduced labor demand due to collapse of employment opportunities that resulted in changes in public policy. Many workers chose early retirement rather than unemployment or were effectively coerced into retirement by a hostile labor market. New employment and pension measures such as preretirement benefits in Denmark and Germany and the Job Release Scheme in the United Kingdom were developed to encourage early retirement (Walker 2006).

Walker (2006: 64) believes that the increased number of people engaging in early retirement from the labor force has "reconstructed old age from a simple age-related status with a single entry point into a much broader category that stretches from around age 50 to death." This has resulted in:

...widespread functional separation of the third (50–74) and fourth (75+) ages, the young-old and the old-old, a distinction that first appeared in France in the 1960s. It has also meant...that public pension systems are no longer the key regulators of retirement. The traditional pattern of labor-force exit at pension age has become a minority one – for example, in Germany (former FDR) and the United Kingdom only around one-third of male entrants to the public pension system come directly from employment.

(Walker 2006: 64)

Walker (2006: 64) also believes that growth of early retirement from the labor force has:

...reinforced the devaluation of older people in the labor market. The downward redefinition of aging has had consequences for the ways that employers perceive older workers and in turn the chances they offer them for reemployment. Indeed, there is a large body of evidence in different E.U. countries to show that third agers are frequently discriminated against with regard to job recruitment, promotions, and training (Drury, 1993, 1997; Walker, 1997). This is despite the fact that age is not a good proxy for the ability to work and learn; therefore discrimination is not only unjust but wasteful of economic capacity and potential. Anecdotal evidence suggests that anti-age discrimination legislation in the United States is a factor in the higher employment rate among older U.S. citizens compared to their non-U.S. counterparts.

During this phase, the social meaning of aging changed from association with pension ages to labor market criteria driven by public policy. Aging came to be seen as an economic problem despite the fact that early retirement was previously seen as a solution to unemployment. According to Walker (2006: 65), extremely pessimistic neoclassical assumptions about the "burden" of aging predominated in economic policy decisions during this time period, and this was a precursor of neoliberal globalization.

Globalization did not yet have the decisive impact on the spread of neoliberal ideas, including aging policy, that it would during the next phase. However, this trend could be anticipated in two Organization for Economic Cooperation and Development reports in the late 1980s and subsequent documents. These included a "'burden of aging' discourse and advocated policy prescriptions that involved a reduction in pay-as-you-go and private/occupational defined-benefit pension schemes and an increase in private, defined contribution ones." However, among European nations only the United Kingdom pursued this policy prescription wholeheartedly at this time, and neoliberal advice was followed closely by former communist bloc countries that were being advised by international governmental organizations such as the World Bank. Walker notes the existence of structural lag between institutional changes and social and cultural changes; during this period, new grassroots discourses were emerging while public policy discourses were dominated by the deserving model of aging or public burden model (Walker 2009: 79).

In the late 1980s and early 1990s, direct political participation by older people increased in many nations:

> Such action is invariably a minority pursuit but, nonetheless, new or recon-
> stituted movements of older people were seen in Denmark, Germany, and the
> United Kingdom while, in 1992, the Italian pensioner party, the oldest of its
> kind in Europe, had its first representative elected to the regional government
> in Rome. A year later, seven pensioner representatives were elected to the
> Dutch parliament (Walker & Naegele, 1999). The character of the political
> and policy discourses emanating from these social movements was, of course,
> fundamentally different from the public policy discourses. In contrast to the
> latter, the grassroots movements emphasized human (including welfare)
> rights, participation, social inclusion, and fierce opposition to age discrimi-
> nation regardless of whether it was blatant or benign.
>
> (Walker 2009: 79)

In the third phase, the assumption that old age is a "burden" on society has resulted in attempts by governments to reduce economic costs of pensions, health, and social services for older adults. The key architects of the neoliberal response to globalization, the World Bank, the International Monetary Fund (IMF), and the World Trade Organization (WTO) have promoted greater personal responsibility and reduced state provisions of retirement benefits. Consistent with their policies, Germany and the United Kingdom made decisions to increase retirement ages, and formulae for pensions were changed in Italy and Sweden to introduce an element of prefunding. The pension reforms in the United Kingdom during the Thatcher administration reconstructed pensions into private pension schemes. This policy increased risks of future deprivation and poverty for some people due to reduction in state pension provision, and the change from public to private pensions has made workers' future pension income more problematic, especially for women who are employed in part-time work (Walker 2006: 66).

Walker (2006) believes that individualization and privatization of pensions is part of a broader trend in which nations are expecting individuals and families to assume risks that were previously considered the collective responsibility of members of the state. The trend has been especially strong in Central and Eastern Europe, driven by the World Bank, and in the United Kingdom and the Southern hemisphere. Walker (2006) believes that there are four reasons why established European welfare states are experiencing a trend toward individualization and privatization of pensions: (1) the belief that globalization and the Transatlantic Consensus that globalization contributes to increased inequality and the need to minimize social costs (Walker 2002); (2) pressures on European pension systems; (3) the argument that social insurance systems created in the early 1900s can no longer be relevant; and (4) the argument that deterioration of structures of early modernity opens new opportunities for human agency in societies in which people follow many different life course patterns. Beck's (1992) and Giddens's (1994) risk society thesis is that calculable risks in industrial society become incalculable and unpredictable in risk society and therefore require changes in basic foundations of modernity such as social security and the nation state in globalized markets.

As a critical theorist, in 2006 Walker (2006: 66–7) provided the following responses to these concerns. Regarding the first argument, he asserted that European welfare states compete well internationally and that there is little evidence that inequality is an inevitable result of globalization. However, fear of global competition may be driving some of the policy agenda, and this can be difficult to distinguish from politicians' concerns about the effects of direct taxation on elections. In response to the second argument, Walker writes that population aging is not the only contributor to the problem but that its combination with early departure from the labor market has contributed to the current situation. Thirdly, Walker responds that the argument that social insurance systems created in the early 1900s can no longer be relevant lacks evidence. He suggests that late-modern working life is characterized by increased employment insecurity, especially for women, and that this trend is likely to increase. Therefore, risk pooling may be more relevant than in the past because increased insecurity makes it less likely that workers will be able to save the money to fund private pensions.

Fourthly, Walker responds to Beck's (1992) and Giddens's (1994) functional analysis that emphasizes reconstruction of the welfare state in response to globalized ecological, scientific, and technological risks. Identifying the welfare state as designed to respond to "external" risks such as unemployment and retirement, considered "accidents of fate," Giddens (1994: 24) suggests that new "manufactured" risks renders the institutions of the welfare state obsolete. However, Walker responds that there is very little or no evidence that existing welfare states cannot continue to address continuing risks such as unemployment and retirement and accommodate new risks.

Critical analysis of development of the "American seniors' movement"

Frank T.Y. Wang's (1999) critical analysis of the "American seniors' movement," social movements by and on behalf of older persons in the U.S. to improve the well-being of older adults, is informed by the Foucauldian model of power/ subject/resistance and addresses gerontological social activism from a political economy perspective. According to Wang (1999: 189), in the United States old age is devalued, and older adults are inevitably perceived as a dependent and useless "other." Old age is pathologized as a social problem, and the negative public image organizes all levels of social life for younger and older people. The negative image has provided a focus for resistance in the seniors' movement, and older people have become active participants in shaping and transforming the ways that they are represented in public discussions. Wang suggests that the dialectical relationship between agent and structure, subject and object, and power and resistance embedded in constant, endless, struggles that is portrayed in Foucault's (1982) model of subject/power/resistance is illustrated by the American seniors' movement in which neither side completely controls the other.

Wang (1999: 190) has made Foucault's notion of power and resistance explicit in relation to experiences of older adults through a reinterpretation of elders' movements in the United States. He demonstrated how socioeconomic and political conditions in specific historical periods shaped identities and strategies of these groups. According to Wang (1999), there are two rationales for addressing this topic. First, common use of Foucault's concept of disciplinary power reinforces the idea of total control of disciplinary power, resulting in the conclusion that power and oppression are inevitable in societies and that escape is impossible. Consideration of Foucault's notion of resistance and subjectivity in which he refers to exercise of power through construction of individuals as subjects has been neglected, resulting in distortion and incompleteness of Foucault's critical project. Intent upon explaining actions of participants in the seniors' movements who have successfully challenged social institutions and created societal changes, Wang (1999: 190) has written that:

> The overemphasis on power and neglecting the subjectivity of Foucault's concepts of power tend to lead to the conclusion that disciplinary power produces social control. This reduces Foucault's approach to a simple

functionalist and instrumentalist account of modern institutions. What has been overlooked are the productive and positive aspects of power that maximize the lives of people. Simplistic use of Foucault's notions of power denies us access to an appreciation of the local experiences and struggles of people around us and denies us chances to learn from Foucault so that we can explore new strategies for social changes.

Wang's (1999) second rationale for addressing the seniors' movements from a Foucauldian perspective is related to Cohen's (1985) strategy-oriented and identity-oriented paradigms of analysis of social movements. He considers the identity-oriented paradigm preferable for understanding actions by older adults in social movements organized to address needs of older people in the U.S. Comparing the identity-oriented paradigm to the strategy-oriented paradigm, Wang (1999: 191) states:

> ... the identity-oriented paradigm seeks to understand subjective experiences of social movements, such as the origin and logic of group solidarity and their search for identity, autonomy, and recognition. Indeed, the formation of collective identity in a social movement is decisive for later interpretations of individual and collective interests and potential strategies for mobilizing the public. Though both types of analysis investigate the vital aspects of social movements, they tend to be mutually exclusive (Cohen 1985). Foucault's notion of subjectivity and power (1982), establishing a dialectic relationship and thus blurring the distinction between agent and structure, offers an alternative analytical framework that is sensitive to the complexity of their reflexive relationship and offers the possibility of closing the gap between the two different paradigms for the study of social movements.

Wang (1999) considers Foucault's concepts of power, subject, and resistance to be major contributions to understanding exercise and response to power, particularly the importance of subjectivity's position at the center of power technology. Foucault identified two types of power: power that operates through repression of subjectivity and, alternatively, power that he considered most effective: power that promotes, cultivates, and nurtures subjectivity. Disciplinary power that represses subjectivity imposes force while producing "truths" for people and hiding "the Truth" (Wang 1999: 191). Wang (1999) explains that in the alternative form of power, acceptance of power occurs by permeating and producing pleasure, discourse, and knowledge, indirectly constituting subjectivity of individuals. This newer form of power influences thought and availability of choices through politics but never achieves total domination. This form shapes identities and regulates views of the world, and power induces participation. The newer form depends on elders' participation in the discourse offered and regulated by power. Participation develops in a way unanticipated by power.

Consistent with the Foucauldian approach emphasizing subjectivities and development of identities through discourse, Wang (1999: 194) advocates exploration of the ways that public discourse shapes our understanding of later adulthood from an historical perspective, as well as the need to question representations of older people. The concept of old age is reshaped over time by competing claims that are often contradictory. In this critical approach, old age is a product of social interaction, culturally and socially given, rather than an individual biological phenomenon. As Walker has indicated, at the beginning of the twentieth century, in industrializing societies that were experiencing a change from values emphasizing traditional authority to greater emphasis on achievement, older adults began to be viewed and represented more negatively and old age more stigmatized. A reinterpretation of old age occurred as the capitalist economy developed, and retirement became institutionalized as a market mechanism to move older people out of the labor market and ensure entry of physically stronger young people into the labor market. As old age came to be seen as a social problem, ageism resulted from the negative discourse about old age, but from a Foucaldian perspective it also made old age a subject for older adults and others to address and redefine. Wang suggests that this negative public discourse about old age contributed to the U.S. seniors' movement.

First generation seniors' movements

Foucault believed that different, including contradictory, discourses can exist within the same strategy and that different strategies can have the same discourse. Discussing the first generation of seniors' movements during the 1930s and 1940s in the U.S., Wang identifies the California Institute of Social Welfare (CISW) and the Townsend group as separate movements that responded to the discourse of old age emphasizing frailty and dependency in different ways. The CISW advocated for increased public assistance for older adults by broadcasting a negative image of older adults as frail and dependent. Its founder, George McLain, organized CISW through his role as a radio show host, and financial support from members helped to support the organization's office, lobbying, and McLain's radio programs. CISW efforts resulted in California ballot initiatives for more public assistance for older adults and fewer bureaucratic challenges to obtain assistance (Wang 1999).

In contrast, Dr. Francis Townsend was a physician and social reformer who offered a view of old age as positive although he also considered older people to be dependent. He emphasized that older adults should be considered legitimate recipients of assistance and recommended that every older person receive $200 to spend each month. Older people were assigned a role to save the U.S. economy since this plan was intended to help end the Great Depression of the 1930s while also meeting financial needs of older people. The Townsend movement achieved widespread support as a political phenomenon with a dues-paying membership of hundreds of thousands of people (Wang 1999).

According to Wang (1999), the successes and demise of both movements were inherent in their simultaneously enabling and limiting discourses. Consistent with ideas proposed by Foucault, Wang (1999) suggests that each discourse is simultaneously enabling and limiting because human beings experience new subjectivity in each specific discursive practice, and they are simultaneously turned into objects constrained by each discourse's norms and logic. The CISW image of older adults as dependent and needy garnered support for assistance to this population, but CISW was discredited in 1948 when the organization demanded that California's first state welfare director be a CISW trustee. Business groups and newspapers responded that if old people were dependent and needy, it was illogical that they would acquire power. McLain was labeled as power hungry and using older adults for personal gain.

The Townsend Movement resulted in the Townsend Plan legislation that was defeated in the U.S. Congress, and this plan was replaced by the Social Security Act passed by Congress in 1935. According to Holtzman (1963, in Wang 1999), the movement's strong identification with Townsend and failure to develop a grassroots structure encouraging participation of its membership was contradictory to its emphasis on the positive role of older people. Confidence in the movement was undermined by public belief that its founders had benefited from it financially (Wang 1999).

Second generation seniors' movements

The demise of the Townsend Movement and passage of the Social Security Act provided the foundation for the second generation seniors' movement. The Townsend Plan focused public debate on consideration of the right of older adults to participate in social change and their right to income. Age was proposed as the borderline between work and retirement, but a long history in the paid labor market was also required for benefits, disqualifying women's labor at home and reinforcing labor market inequalities (Wang 1999).

Second generation movements in the 1950s were focused on members' shared status as retired workers, and emerging groups included the National Association of Retired Civil Employees (NARCE) and National Retired Teachers' Association (NRTA) that became the American Association of Retired Persons (AARP). Wang notes that these developments reflected a shift in discourse about old age from a focus on dependence in later adulthood to status as retired worker, illustrating agent and structure, as well as the reflexive relationship of power and resistance. The NRTA hoped to provide material benefits while creating a new and positive definition of old age through a mutual help approach. AARP's emphasis on identity as retired workers was intended to counteract the image of older people as dependent and frail. This new social movement focused on cultural practices of identity and on civil society rather than public policies and the state or economy (Wang 1999). Relating this to Foucault's perspectives, Wang (1999: 201–2) has written:

> The search for one's own claim or identity directly questions current practices of knowledge formation and challenges the privileges of knowledge, in which Foucault sees claims to truth as the center of modern disciplinary power.

The politics of identity is one of the major characters of contemporary struggle against domination. The seniors' movement is no exception.

When Ethel Percy Andrus, the founder of NRTA, persuaded a private insurance
company to provide an inexpensive group health insurance plan to members
in 1955, the subject moved beyond abstraction into practice. A policy of this
type had not been available to people with a group identification as "old" but
now became available to people belonging to a "retired" group. Wang suggests
that gender discrimination in the labor market may have been the foundation
of group solidarity for teachers and influenced the founding of NRTA although
women's issues were not the stated focus of this organization. Andrus may
not have considered feminist discourse to be an effective counterdiscourse in
response to her concerns when receiving her first pension check, but she identified mass organization as a strategy for gaining a voice in pluralist politics in the
U.S. Wang's Foucauldian perspective emphasizes that her perception of the
discourses available to her was limited by the structures surrounding her, including pluralist politics, the capitalist economy, and the work-achievement-oriented
welfare state. Foucault notes that "the aim of struggles is the power and so people
focus on the "immediate enemy" rather than the "chief enemy" (Foucault 1982:
211). The low level of pensions was the immediate enemy, while the chief enemy
was the patriarchal relations in the labor market (Wang 1999).

Third generation seniors' movements

These organizations provided the foundation for the third round of seniors' movements, and the new generation of movements emphasized increased political
participation. AARP demonstrated that later adulthood can be rewarding, and this
helped many older adults and members of younger cohorts to recognize age as
the foundation for a shared identity of old age. During the 1970s and 1980s,
seniors' groups increased their power to influence public policies, with preexisting groups becoming politicized while militant groups were established. They
demanded positive recognition of old age by society, and the Gray Panthers was
the most vocal group. Maggie Kuhn, the group's founder, addressed discrimination against both young and old by middle aged people and drew an intergenerational membership, while maintaining its orientation as a seniors' movement
organization (Wang 1999).

In the third round, AARP has grown and expanded services to members. It
no longer speaks only on behalf of retired workers but attempts to represent the
interests of older adults in general. Following the death of Andrus in 1967, AARP
initiated efforts to influence public policy through lobbying and government
linkages but remained a moderate organization primarily attracting middle-class
and professional retirees. In contrast, the membership of the National Council of
Senior Citizens (NCSC) is strongly associated with the union movement and
includes a working-class membership (Wang 1999).

Wang asserts that the dramatic success of seniors' movements in achieving financial support, symbolic recognition, and political access resulted in an era of intergenerational conflict in the 1980s. Furthermore, the power of older adults has been exaggerated by the media and has contributed to conflicts regarding intergenerational equity. The trend toward negative views of older adults as a group has required advocacy organizations, including older members and advocates on behalf of older adults, to work to protect older adults' status (Wang 1999).

Wang (1999) considers Foucault's idea of tactical use of discourses in different strategies to be relevant in the intergenerational conflict debate. He believes that this debate has been possible because of successes of older adults' groups in the 1970s and 1980s. Consistent with Walker's (2006) assertions regarding intergenerational conflict, Wang asserts that this debate reflects socially constructed reality in an era of fiscal constraint.

Wang does not attribute the intergenerational conflict debate only to successes of older adults' groups. Consistent with Walker's (2006) political economy perspective regarding experiences in European countries, Wang (1999: 207–8) indicates that in the United States:

> ...the rise of intergenerational conflict should be understood as part of the 'welfare state crisis...and the retreat of the state in the social provision of welfare launched by neoconservatives who came into power in the 1980s.... the idea of intergenerational conflict is socially constructed by the media, politicians, and economists to divert attention from demands for government responsibility and universal entitlement programs....By framing aging issues as a conflict between the young and the old, the role of the state disappears, and the once public responsibility of social care for the elderly is reprivatized. Despite the negative portrayal of the elderly as 'greedy geezers,' opinion polls seem to suggest that the elderly are perceived as deserving of continued public support (Gilliland and Havir 1990; Coombs and Holladay 1995). Although intergenerational conflict has not marginalized the needs of the elderly, lawmakers may no longer assume the needs and legitimacy of the elderly, or, at minimum, their needs may become secondary to budget concerns (Estes 1989).

Wang (1999) also addresses the class-based nature of the American seniors' movement. The interests of working-, middle-, and upper-class elderly can be represented through AARP and NCSC, but political underrepresentation persists for more disadvantaged elderly, including minority elderly, women, and poor older adults. According to Wang, AARP and NCSC have not paid adequate attention to social and economic conditions of severely disadvantaged older adults.

Writing in 1999, Wang suggested that the American seniors' movement had reached its limits as a result of entering an era of fiscal restraints and growth of the older population. Older adults continued to be active agents in resisting the effects of the negative image of old age, but they were forced to pit themselves against each other. They are active agents in efforts to construct counterdiscourses and resist the effects of the negative image of old age, but their freedom of choice to form group identity is constrained by the social structure. Paid employment continues to be deeply cultivated as a way of evaluating oneself and others, and the legacy of the second generation of older adult movements in which paid employment was perceived as the only viable way of defending deserving status in later adulthood has continued. Wang (1999: 2008) considered this to be an example of Foucault's supposition that "Each discourse is simultaneously enabling and limiting," and this implies that inevitably there will be exclusion.

Foucault advocated use of multiple points of resistance that are present everywhere in the power network since he did not believe that there could be universal social transformation. Contemporary older adults' movements in the United States have not transformed the fundamental social structure or promoted the well-being of all older adults during a time of fiscal constraint, but they have transformed the negative discourse on aging into one of worker identity and political participation. Wang suggests that the seniors' movement is a neverending struggle in which current counterdiscourse usually becomes the central discourse in the future (Wang 1999).

Wang (1999) views patterns of resistance as culturally dependent and suggests that in a liberal democratic capitalist society like the U.S. formation of organized special interest groups to engage in the political process is a normative and socially accepted approach to resistance. However, not all groups have the power to access this hierarchically distributed form of resistance. Many immigrant elders come from societies without histories of civil participation and organizing and also lack attributes such as wealth, verbal ability, professional expertise and time for organizing groups. Wang (1999) points out that minority elderly, female elderly, and poor elderly have participated marginally in seniors' movements in the United States.

Alternative forms of resistance by older people

Critical theory supports the idea that history and social context influence the forms of expression of resistance. In the U.S., pluralist interest group politics has provided the context for collective efforts by older adults to resist oppression, engage in a politics of identity, and gain access to decision making. In his discussion of suicide by older Chinese women, Wang provides a contrasting cultural example of older adults' resistance to domination. He considers suicide by older Chinese women to be a local form of resistance that is consistent with Foucault's belief that there is power in all social relations, including everyday social relations. Wang believes that although this form of resistance may be considered abnormal or deviant by professionals, suicide by older Chinese women is an action that is as significant as civil organizing as an attempt to change power relations. He suggests that suicide by an elderly Chinese woman is equally meaningful as an effort to change power relations in her life as an older adult's participation in the Gray Panthers in the United States. Historical and local contexts must be known in order to fully understand the meaning of resistance for specific individuals (Wang 1999).

Unlike the common Western view of suicide as a mental health problem in which personal behavior expresses interpersonal anger and conflict (Osgood and McIntosh 1986), Wang believes that in Chinese society suicide has a strong social and collective character. Historically, for Chinese women suicide has been a socially acceptable solution to various problems perceived as having no alternative for resolution. Female suicide has been sanctioned by the state through a public ritual of awarding tablets to some women who committed suicide. Wang (1999: 211) sees this ritualized approval as consistent with Foucault's (1977) view that:

> any tool of power must involve the issue of representation. Through the power of naming, the state was able to normalize certain behaviors and marginalize others. The effects of awarding the tablets were not targeted at the deceased but the living. The tablets make the behavior of suicide visible to other women and serve as a 'model' to discipline the whole social body.

Wang continues:

> The state-promoted discourse of suicide offers a subject for Chinese women and a real tool in their struggle to change power relations. For these women, committing suicide was not a 'hegemony' that showed that they were cheated or hidden from the truth but a real choice that could grant them not only termination of their suffering but also the power, the means, to punish others…. In the context of Chinese culture…the act of senior suicide itself convicts the children, especially sons and daughters-in-law, of the most immoral crimes, unfilial behavior (Wolf 1975). Chinese women can replicate the discourse of suicide not because they are deceived from identifying the 'real' source of their oppression, the patriarchal Chinese family system, but because the discourse produces a subject that can dramatically alter the power relations.
>
> (Wang 1999: 211–12)

Critically oriented activism: Maggie Kuhn and the Gray Panthers

Within the context of civic participation in pluralist interest group politics in the U.S., activism in the third generation seniors' movements was initiated by Maggie Kuhn, a civil rights and anti-Vietnam War activist, after she experienced mandatory retirement at age 65. Collaborating with retired friends, Kuhn founded the Gray Panthers coalition that brought older people and youth together to address the need for basic social and economic changes in the political system. Kuhn (1987: 378) wrote about her reactions to retirement and beginning the Gray Panthers' organization:

In 1970, when I faced mandatory retirement at the age of 65, I was anxious and depressed. I was leaving a job that I loved for an isolated retirement, caring for my 90-year-old mother, who was wheelchair-bound by arthritis, and a 60-year-old brother with many emotional problems. They were financially and emotionally dependent on me. With reduced income and without the support of professional colleagues, I felt bereft.

To ease my anxiety, I wrote a memo to five of my friends who were in a similar situation, asking this question: 'What do we do with the rest of our lives?' As we met to consider this question, it was clear that we needed one another to regroup our lives and that we were at a juncture of life when we could begin something new. We could take risks together in our own supportive community. We could reach out to others and organize for change. We could be risk takers with nothing to lose but our fears and isolation!

Although she was not formally educated as a critical gerontologist, Kuhn's professional and personal experiences led her to believe by the age of 65 that it was only through broad-based social changes addressing issues affecting the entire society that the needs of older adults would be met with justice, equity, and compassion (Kuhn 1987). Social justice for people of all ages and all social classes was included in Gray Panthers' organizational goals from the beginning. Kuhn urged that "'we who are old...build coalitions, and close ranks between the disadvantaged groups...contending for small slivers of power. [We] have the responsibility to transcend our personal needs and [work] for a just and humane society that puts people first'" (Sanjek 2009: 245). In 1978, at a Gray Panthers National Steering Committee meeting, the following principles were approved:

1. We are NOT a vested interest group for the elderly.
2. We are NOT out to win points for older people at the expense of other groups.
3. We ARE a movement comprised of all ages dedicated to changing people's attitudes about aging.
4. We ARE a movement dedicated to improving the quality of life for all people.

(Sanjek 2009: 155)

Because they were strongly committed to civic participation, Kuhn and other members of the Gray Panthers advocated for a "Gray Power" goal of "mobilization of older Americans to heal and humanize our society and make society safe for their survivors" (Kuhn 1987: 378). Kuhn's views were consistent with those of the Frankfurt theorists who believed that instrumental reason unreflectively supports effective means for any accepted purpose, and she was critical of the abuses of technocratic thinking that dominated industrialization and administration in the United States. The Gray Panthers' and other advocates' responses to abuses, according to Kuhn, were activism in:

reaching out to organize the victims of our economic system and enlist and empower them for the public interest as well as their own! A safe, just, and peaceful world is the legacy that we seek for those who will come after us. That's the transcending Gray Power that our hate-torn world desperately needs.

(Kuhn 1987: 378)

Consistent with critical gerontology, Kuhn (1987: 376) attributed many difficulties experienced by older adults to structural causes and was concerned about the biomedicalization of aging:

Issues pertaining to old age and aging constitute an enormous challenge to the whole society and raise basic moral and ethical questions about social justice and the survival of our society. The problems of age are basically societal, not merely personal and individualistic. Most of us live highly private lives with family and close friends, failing to see ourselves as social beings personally imprinted by the people we live and work with, powerfully conditioned by social class and the economic forces that shape our attitudes, feelings, and behavior. These forces victimize us or empower us. They pre-dispose us to health and well-being or to sickness of mind, body, and spirit.

Instead of seeing the issue of age in a societal context, we view the aging process as one of foreordained personal degradation tied to a biological clock. Medically, we often distinguish between the young-old (65–74 years), the old (75–84 years), and the old-old (85 and over). These are statistical time cycles for the appearance of multiple chronic ailments or terminal diseases. We view these as *personal*, individual problems. Rarely do we see them in relation to the issues of society and its stresses and hazards.

Consistent with critical gerontology's goal of identification of possibilities for emancipatory social change and positive ideals for later life, Maggie Kuhn and the Gray Panthers worked to change structures of domination. Their goals were consistent with a structural approach to define and achieve a meaningful context for later adulthood that can help to guide individual aging, inform institutional and policy responses, and penetrate ageism. Kuhn (1987) valued the contributions of sociologist Carroll Estes and her colleagues to theory and research addressing political economy of aging.

Maggie Kuhn and the Gray Panthers addressed a very broad range of issues up to the time of her death in 1995 at age 89. These included activism to eliminate mandatory retirement practices in public and private employment, opposition to the Vietnam War, advocacy for reductions in military spending, advocacy for physical and mental health care including patients' rights and universal health care through a national health service, support for reproductive freedom (legal abortion), advocacy for intergenerational housing programs, support for National Public Radio, nursing home reform, advocacy for an Equal Rights Amendment to the Constitution of the United States in order to protect women's rights, anti-poverty efforts, and advocacy for environmental protection.

A major coalescing issue in the early years of the Gray Panthers movement was the issue that motivated Maggie Kuhn to establish the Gray Panthers, mandatory retirement from paid employment. The sequence of events that began with the conflict between Kuhn's desire to continue employment and her mandatory retirement supported by federal policy resulted in elimination of legalized mandatory retirement on the basis of age in most jobs in the U.S. This provides an example of the critical dialectic that an idea or event generates its opposite, leading to a reconciliation of opposites. Kuhn and the Gray Panthers resisted policies enacted by those in power and achieved reconciliation. They used civic participation and available political opportunities to empower themselves and create lasting changes in social structures. Power relations were altered.

In the U.S., since the 1880s employers had begun to implement mandatory retirement policies at a predetermined age. Sanjek (2009: 3) writes that by the 1920s and 1930s, older people, as well as African Americans and women, were a second class or reserve army of the working class. They were unable to participate fully as income earners because employers would arbitrarily assess their appropriateness for employment based on perceptions of efficiency, tractability, or age. Their "exclusion became even more entrenched after Social Security helped make an exit at age sixty-five obligatory in most workplaces. (In 1890 three-quarters of white men over sixty-five still worked, in 1920 60 percent did; by 1970 only one-quarter were employed, while a similar number preferred but were not allowed to continue working)" (Sanjek 2009: 3–4).

The initial Gray Panther success in changing retirement policy was in California, where members lobbied state representatives for abolition of mandatory retirement. In 1976, Governor Brown signed legislation: "allowing employees to continue working irrespective of age as long as they met competence standards approved by the California Industrial Welfare Commission. While other states had similar laws for public workers, California was first to include the private sector" (Sanjek 2009: 76). Likewise, as a result of persuasion by Gray Panthers in Philadelphia in 1976, the member of Congress from that city introduced congressional legislation to eliminate age 65 as the upper limit of federal age discrimination protection. Congressional and state testimonies by Gray Panthers followed, and the process moved quickly:

> President Carter was on record opposing mandatory retirement, and [federal] Commissioner of Aging Arthur Flemming, seventy-two, a longtime friend of Maggie, launched a 'crusade' against it....Congressional proposals were consolidated in a bill by Representative Claude Pepper, seventy-seven, to eliminate mandatory retirement for most federal workers and raise the private sector retirement age to seventy...When it passed and it was signed by Carter in 1978, Maggie declared, 'Our struggle is hardly over,' and called for full abolition of mandatory retirement.
>
> (Sanjek 2009: 145–6)

The Panthers continued their activism to change federal policy, and mandatory retirement was eliminated in 1986 in most private sector employment when the legislation was passed by Congress and signed into law by President Ronald Reagan when he was 75.

Since Maggie Kuhn's death, the Gray Panthers have continued to be active despite fundraising challenges. Activism has focused on many social, health, and economic issues including defense of Social Security and Medicare and opposition to Wall Street commercial interests' proposals to privatize Social Security and use Social Security payroll taxes to create private investment accounts for individuals. Members have advocated broadening Social Security payroll taxes so that the earning cap is eliminated and all earned income will be subject to the Social Security tax. The Gray Panthers have advocated for pharmaceutical companies to make generic equivalent medications more available. They have opposed President George W. Bush's 2001 proposal for tax reductions for earners with the highest incomes, corporate fraud, and the U.S. invasion of Iraq (Sanjek 2009).

Many of these issues still exist in the U.S., and Gray Panthers' biographer Roger Sanjek, who became involved with the organization as a post-graduate student in California in 1977, believes that the organization's future will continue to be tied to the larger progressive movement of interconnected political groups in the U.S. Activist groups are linked to others, and organizations thrive when many people become indignant and defiant, as Maggie Kuhn did. Political energy develops for civic participation, and large organizations such as the Gray Panthers develop. Sanjek (2009: 350) asserts: "As goes the liberal, progressive, left spectrum within American political life, so will go the Gray Panthers". He concludes: "Whether or not the Gray Panthers survive or flourish, the world of the twenty-first century will require something like them. Future political activists, young or old, will not need to reinvent the Gray Panthers' view of the human life cycle, their concept of the person, their array of tactics, or their intergenerationalism. What they will need is a readiness, as Maggie urged, to 'get out there and do something about injustice'" (Sanjek 2009: 252).

Summary

Critical theory in gerontology is influenced primarily by the work of first generation Frankfurt School theorists Theodor Adorno and Max Horkheimer, second generation theorist Jurgen Habermas, and by Michel Foucault's post-structuralist theoretical perspectives. It focuses on criticism of the process of power, and in contemporary social gerontology critical perspectives are driven by concern and include political economy of aging, feminist gerontology, humanistic gerontology, theories of diversity, and specific social constructionist approaches. Postmodern trends that resulted in demand for a critical approach to gerontology include biomedicalization of gerontology, the generational equity debate, the mood of cost containment, and nostalgia for positive images of old age amid awareness that there is more to aging than is reflected in the disease model of aging.

Jecker suggested that critical theory makes room for other perspectives by questioning, enlarging, and unifying. Moody thinks that critical theory should be used to examine and understand structures of domination and change strategies with the goal of creating spaces in which there is potential for emancipation from domination.

The two patterns of study in critical gerontology have been humanistic dimensions of aging and structural components of aging. The political economy perspective posits that economic dependency is not primarily the result of chronological age but results from relationships principally between age and labor market and age and the welfare state that are socially constructed. In the political economy perspective, characteristics such as gender, race, and class are considered pivotal variables in aging because they predetermine a person's location in the social order.

Wang's critical analysis of the "American seniors' movement" and alternative forms of resistance by older Chinese women and others is informed by Foucault's model of power/subject/resistance. Maggie Kuhn and the Gray Panthers worked to change structures of domination in the third wave of movements by and on behalf of older people. They created major achievements through approaches that were consistent with critical theorists' structural approach to define and achieve a meaningful context for later adulthood that can help to guide individual aging, inform institutional and policy responses, and penetrate ageism.

5 Feminist gerontology

Key concepts

1. Feminist theory is a multidisciplinary area of critical theory with origins in civil rights and women's liberation movements that questioned the status quo during the last half of the twentieth century.

2. Origins of feminist perspectives in sociology also include the influence of social constructionist and other postmodern approaches.

3. Feminists deconstruct ideas, theories, and methods in order to understand their meaning, and they view knowledge as socially situated.

4. Theoretical developments in the 1970s that were based on scholars' study that emphasized differences between men and women became problematic because of overgeneralization about each gender.

5. A stage of feminist thinking about gender grounded in diversity of experiences has existed since the mid-1980s, and this perspective views women and men in terms of relationships to social structure and the relational character of gender.

6. In feminist gerontology, opportunities and constraints related to gender and age are examined at individual, interactional, and institutional levels, including attention to the aging of gendered selves, exploration of diverse cultural expectations for people of different ages and genders, and age and gender specific rules for distribution of material items and resources.

7. Socialist feminist theories of aging are based on the belief that problematic life circumstances of older women have resulted from patriarchal and race-based definitions of the reproductive and productive activities acceptable for women and men that have resulted in women's and men's different retirement experiences.

8. The feminist political economy of aging perspective aims to understand how vulnerability and dependency of women throughout their lives is rendered by dominant social institutions, particularly economic and political systems.

9. Feminist theories and research about men's lives result from understanding of the importance of gendered power relationships and the view that both

femininity and masculinity need to be viewed as social constructs that change over time within cultural and national contexts.

10. Robert Meadows and Kate Davidson assert that attention to the lives of old men provides insights into critical axes of inequality through which old men are subordinated, especially in relation to younger men.

Introduction

Chapter 5 provides an introduction to feminist theory and explanation of theoretical perspectives in feminist gerontology, with particular emphasis on socialist feminist theories and feminist political economy theories of aging. Robert Meadows' and Kate Davidson's feminist analysis of maintenance of manliness in later life by older men who were interviewed in a British research study is described with particular emphasis on issues related to hegemonic masculinities.

Foundations of feminist theory

Feminist theory is an interdisciplinary area of critical theory with origins in feminist movements of the 1800s and earlier 1900s and civil rights and women's liberation movements that questioned the status quo during the last half of the twentieth century. Origins of feminist perspectives in sociology also include the influence of social constructionist and other postmodern approaches. Consistent with social constructionism, feminists deconstruct ideas, theories, and methods in order to understand their meanings, and they address the reality that knowledge is socially situated (Allen and Walker 2009: 522).

Theoretical developments proceeded in the 1970s with scholars' study of women in society that emphasized differences between men and women, but this was problematic because this focus led to overgeneralization. Each gender was essentialized and treated as a homogeneous category (Baca Zinn et al. 2007). In the 1970s, the feminist idea that femininity and subordination of women is a social construction led to exploration of the social construction of masculinity and men's power (Baca Zinn et al. 2007).

In the next wave of feminism, some women claimed that the feminist view of universal sisterhood marginalized or failed to acknowledge their major concerns. When "gender" was used as a generic category in order to unify women, it produced divisions among women. Although "the feminist call for women to move out of the kitchen and into the workplace" resonated with many college-educated white women, this:

... seemed absurd or irrelevant to many working-class women and women of color. They were already working for wages, as had many of their mothers and grandmothers, and did not consider access to jobs and public life 'liberating.' For many of these women, liberation had more to do with organizing in communities and workplaces – often alongside men – for better schools, better pay, decent benefits, and other policies to benefit their neighborhoods, jobs, and families. The feminism of the 1970s did not seem to address these issues.... As more and more women analyzed their own experiences, they began to address the power relations that created differences among women and the part that privileged women played in the oppression of others. For many women of color, working-class women, lesbians, and women in contexts outside the United States (especially women in non-Western societies), the focus on male domination was a distraction from other oppression.

(Baca Zinn et al. 2007: 149–50)

A stage of feminist thinking about gender grounded in diversity of experiences has existed since the mid-1980s. This perspective views women and men in terms of relationships to social structure and the "relational character of gender" (Connell 1992: 736, in Baca Zinn et al. 2007: 153). Baca Zinn et al. emphasize the importance of addressing the reality that:

... differences *among* women and *among* men are created in the context of structured relationships. Some women derive benefits from their race and class position and from their location in the global economy, while they are simultaneously restricted by gender. In other words, such women are subordinated by patriarchy, yet their relatively privileged positions within hierarchies of race, class, and the global political economy intersect to create for them an expanded range of opportunities, choices, and ways of living. They may even use their race and class advantage to minimize some of the consequences of patriarchy and/or to oppose other women. Similarly, one can become a man in opposition to other men.

(Baca Zinn et al. 2007: 153–4)

Baca Zinn and her colleagues (2007: 151) assert that the power of nation states and the significance of national borders have decreased since the late twentieth century due to increases in transnational trade, international migration, and global systems of production and communication. Global economic restructuring influences gender relations throughout the world: "Decisions made in corporate headquarters located in Los Angeles, Tokyo, or London may have immediate repercussions on how women and men thousands of miles away organize their work, community, and family lives (Sassen, 1991). It is no longer possible to study gender relations without giving attention to global processes and inequalities..." (Baca Zinn et al. 2007: 151–2). Consistent with political economy theory, Baca Zinn et al. (2007: 152) elaborate:

Around the world, women's paid and unpaid labor is key to global development strategies. Yet it would be a mistake to conclude that gender is molded from the 'top down.' What happens on a daily basis in families and workplaces simultaneously constitutes and is constrained by structural transnational institutions. For instance, in the second half of the twentieth century young, single women, many of them from poor rural areas, were (and continue to be) recruited for work in export assembly plants along the U.S.-Mexico border, in East and Southeast Asia, in Silicon Valley, in the Caribbean, and in Central America. While the profitability of these multinational factories depends, in part, on management's ability to manipulate young women's ideologies of gender, the women...do not respond passively or uniformly, but actively resist, challenge, and accommodate.

Toni Calasanti (2009: 473) explains that theories of gender relations clarify realities such as the fact that privilege can be harmful and subordinate status can result in strengths:

> ...women's immersion in the work of daily life, including kin keeping, provide them resources in later life that men may not enjoy at that stage. Not only do such networks offer social support in old age; for those with fewer material resources, such networks may also ensure a decent quality of life. Because men are not responsible for domestic life, they often access social networks through their wives. Thus, some men can be highly dependent on their wives for social and material resources, and men who are not married often have smaller networks.

Feminist theorists also point out that opportunities for human agency result from social stratification and that political theorizing leading to social changes is needed. Social changes by and on behalf of women are core incentives for feminist theorizing (Allen and Walker 2009). Jessie Bernard (1972) provided an important foundation in family studies for moving beyond traditional theories of family roles. She studied gender inequality in heterosexual marriage and demonstrated that gender neutrality in families was a myth. Bernard found that relationships were composed of "his" and "hers," and subsequent feminist research challenged assumptions about motherhood as a woman's calling and men as breadwinners and women as caregivers. Normative approaches that idealized the nuclear family did not explain diversity in women's lives and family structures. Realities in many families challenged the idealized norm. For example, many working-class women and women of color have been both breadwinners and caregivers, and not all women have wanted to become mothers (Allen and Walker 2009: 520–1, 524).

In the twenty-first century, there are many variations of feminist theory. These range from the perspective that gender is a key organizing principle to the perspective that gender is interconnected with race, class, sexual orientation, and age with which it intersects. However, in contemporary feminist thought there is a shared assumption that social stratifications of gender, race, class, sexual orientation and other attributes are intersecting influences that combine in unique ways in people's lives (Allen and Walker 2009: 521).

Development of feminist gerontology

In feminist gerontology, opportunities and constraints related to gender and age are examined at individual, interactional, and institutional levels. This includes attention to the aging of gendered selves, exploration of diverse cultural expectations for people of different ages and genders, and age and gender specific rules for distribution of resources and material items (Allen and Walker 2009). However, before the 1980s, there was little explicit attention among gerontological scholars to experiences of older women. At that time, some feminist scholars began to question lack of attention to women in retirement and other research. Sociological study in the area of family studies had not included study of older adults since family studies conformed to stereotypes of the "Standard North American Family" with father as breadwinner, stay at home wife, and dependent biological children (Allen and Walker 2009: 519).

Initial responses to concerns about lack of theorizing about older women took the form of including older women in research samples and in models and developing theories based on men's experiences. Often women were assessed against an implicit standard set by men. According to Calasanti (2009: 472):

> Scholars noted differences between men's and women's labor force participation histories and women's subsequent lower retirement benefits but failed to ask why women's work histories were more intermittent, why Social Security rewards stable participation, why dependent spouse benefits amount to only half of the retired worker benefit, or whether women and men garner similar workplace returns for similar human capital attributes.

Calasanti (2009: 472–3) asserts that:

> In its theories of such systems of inequality, feminist gerontology recognizes that both women and men have gender and that their experiences are structured by *gender relations*: dynamic, constructed, institutionalized processes by which people orient their behaviors to ideals of manhood and womanhood, influencing life chances as they do so. Gender is not a biological given but is what people collectively agree that natural sex attributes mean....
>
> Thus, the gender identities that emerge in social interaction also serve to privilege men – give them unearned advantages – while they usually disadvantage women, even as people resist and reformulate seemingly 'natural' differences and meanings.
>
> Gender relations are embedded in patterns of behavior such that they are generally invisible, taken for granted, and unquestioned, as they reflect the way that social institutions, such as paid work or family normally operate. The systematic nature of gender relations means that even though individuals enact them, gender relations are not dependent on any one person's actions or intentions. Because men's privileges are intimately tied to women's

disadvantages, the situation of one group cannot be understood without at least implicit reference to the position of the other.

Critical theory had failed to theorize the relations of inequality underlying gender differences, and emergence of feminist gerontology in the 1990s addressed this need. New theories have been developed from women's perspectives, but feminist gerontology also includes men's perspectives. Calasanti (2009: 471) believes that feminist gerontology contributes to knowledge about aging in general because it theorizes gender relations and addresses experiences of both women and men.

Feminist theorists Katherine Allen and Alexis Walker (2009: 518) believe that knowing women's history and taking a position on where women have been and want to go is important for improving women's lives, lives of older adults, and one's own life. They emphasize authorship of one's own narratives, saying that it is especially important for people with subjugated histories to write their own histories so that they are not written by others. Continued subordination of women, older adults, and people belonging to racial and ethnic minority groups is more likely if group narratives and history are lost.

Socialist feminist theories of aging

Socialist feminist theories of aging are based on the belief that problematic life circumstances of older women have resulted from "patriarchal (and race-based) definitions of the productive and reproductive activities acceptable for women and men and the categorization of skilled and unskilled jobs [that] constituted a basis, expression, and perpetuation of women's subordination and men's domination, resulting in women's and men's different retirement experiences" (Calasanti and Zajicek 1993: 123). Often only paid labor is considered "work," implying that much of women's labor is not "work." Specific theoretical concepts created or revisioned by socialist feminists have changed the direction of gerontological research: "(1) patriarchy and the paradigm of domination; (2) gendering processes within organizations; (3) production and reproduction as delineated by the dialectical relations between private and public spheres; (4) family; and (5) the gendered welfare system" (Calasanti and Zajicek 1993: 120–1).

Socialist feminists describe a "paradigm of domination," a concept that "gender, class, and racial/ethnic relations constitute an interlocking system of oppression" in addition to oppressions resulting from the dialectical relationship between capitalism and patriarchy (Calasanti and Zajicek 1993: 121). Focus on the paradigm of domination is related to the concept of racial formation, "the process by which social, economic and political forces determine the content and importance of racial categories, and by which they are in turn shaped by racial meanings" (Calasanti and Zajicek 1993: 121). Race and ethnicity contribute to differences in the shape and content of patriarchy and class and gender relations (Calasanti and Zajicek 1993). This focus has also included:

a *relational* understanding of the structuring of class, race, and gender [that] can be perceived as social processes through which class and race/ethnicity historically structure the concrete meanings of gender, and simultaneously as processes through which class and race/ethnicity also acquire their specific meaning in the context of gender relations.

(Calasanti and Zajicek 1993: 121–2)

Calasanti (2009: 471) emphasizes that "a focus of intersecting inequalities is critical to understanding those experiences of aging and that feminist geron- tology is uniquely able to offer scholars a lens through which to view these inter- sections." It focuses broadly on intersections of other systems of inequality with age and gender, and the focus on theorizing "the larger system of intersecting relations of inequality" is shared by other groups of scholars driven by social movements including labor, gay and lesbian, civil rights, and the Gray Panthers (Calasanti 2009: 472).

Consistent with discussion of critical theory in Chapter 4, the issue of inter- secting inequalities addressed by feminist gerontologists focuses on power and privilege. Older women's and men's lives are influenced by their positions in hierarchies of racial, ethnic, sexual, and class-based locations. For example, African Americans of both genders have higher poverty rates than Caucasian women, and more women than men are poor. Some feminist gerontological theo- rists have developed criteria to assess systems of privilege and oppression (Calasanti 2009; Young 1990):

Based on these criteria, we might define a group as oppressed to the extent that they experience economic marginalization, powerlessness, and a lack of autonomy and status, and stigmatization. Those who are privileged use their greater resources to control those who are disadvantaged and justify these inequalities through ideologies that deem them to be 'natural' and thus beyond dispute or based on social necessity or the will of a higher power (Calasanti & Slevin, 2006; King, 2006). Recently feminist gerontologists have used these criteria to theorize old age itself as a social location, part of a system of age relations that intersects with other forms of inequality.

(Calasanti 2009: 174)

When the intersections of race, class, and gender are considered in relation to the social institution of the family, there are several points from feminist studies that are relevant to theorizing about the experiences of diverse older adults. Families are not monolithic, and they can be analyzed best by looking at under- lying structures. Actual behavior of the elderly, women, people of color, and children is distorted by the dominant ideology glorifying family; there is more fluidity in boundaries of family, work, and other institutions than previously believed; and the tenacity of race, class, and gender structures and people's efforts to change these systems are apparent in experiences of groups immigrat- ing to the U.S. (Andersen and Collins 2007: 273–4).

An additional intersection of hierarchically ordered personal characteristics is manifested in intersection of age, gender, and sexuality since heterosexuals are advantaged and homosexuals disadvantaged on the basis of sexual orientation. According to Calasanti (2009: 476), in jurisdictions where entitlements such as employee benefits and Social Security and other entitlements are available only to heterosexuals, sexuality is a criteria for privilege and oppression: "To begin, *heteronormality* (norms, beliefs, and practices that naturalize heterosexuality) is a key organizing principle of society (Stein, 2008). That is, the assumption of heterosexuality as natural lies at the heart of social organization, shaping the experiences of people of all sexual preferences." Calasanti (2009: 476) continues:

> ...construction of certain behaviors is social, and as is the case with gender, race, ethnicity, and old age, societies construct heterosexual and nonheterosexual people differently, with those differences both reflecting and perpetuating inequality. Sexuality is thus more than identity...; it is basic to social organization and 'an important focus of power and resistance'
>
> (Heaphy, 2007, p. 194).

An issue in need of further exploration is whether age itself not only exacerbates existing inequalities but confers loss of power even if the older adults have advantages in other social hierarchies. There is continued labor market discrimination against older women in hiring, earnings, and job stability, and older patients more often than younger people become less able to exert control over their bodies when doctors withhold information, services, and treatment (Calasanti 2009: 475).

Gender-based labor practices will affect the experiences of diverse groups of older adults globally for generations to come. Focusing on the United States, Andersen and Collins (2007: 268–69) offer a perspective that is relevant to economic divisions throughout the world that are associated with class, race and gender "resulting in labor and consumer markets that routinely advantage some and disadvantage others....corporate and government structures create jobs for some while leaving others underemployed or without work." A dual labor market exists that includes:

> (1) a primary labor market characterized by relatively high wages, opportunities for advancement, employee benefits, and rules of due process that protect workers' rights; and (2) a secondary labor market (where most women and minorities are located) characterized by low wages, little opportunity for advancement, few benefits, and little protection for workers.
>
> (Andersen and Collins 2007: 269)

The dual labor market results in a persistent wage gap across gender and race even when education is equal, and gender segregation and race segregation intersect (Andersen and Collins 2007: 269). Differences in the retirement opportunities available to women and men have resulted from patriarchal and race-based definitions of activities acceptable for men and women and the categorization of skilled and unskilled jobs (Calasanti and Zajicek 1993).

Andersen and Collins (2007) have also observed that as a result of the intersection of gender segregation and race segregation in the dual labor market in the U.S.:

> women of color are most likely to be working in occupations where most of the other workers are also women of color. At the same time, men of color are segregated into particular segments of the market, too. Indeed, there is a direct connection between gender and racial segregation and wages because [according to the U.S. Department of Labor 2005] wages are lowest in occupations where women of color predominate.
>
> (Andersen and Collins 2007: 269–70)

Disparities in employment opportunities and income earlier in life are reflected in differences in retirement incomes for older people belonging to different races.

Calasanti and Zajicek's (1993) socialist feminist approach to the dialectic between production and reproduction describes interlocking dominations that implicate both men and women in relationships between maintenance (reproduction) and creation (production). Gendered division of labor and gender ideology, in addition to the structure of labor force participation of men and women, results in differences in relationships of men and women to production and reproduction and these structure labor force participation of men and women. This has implications for financial well-being of women as well as men in later adulthood. There is more than one women's standpoint because of the interlocking character of domination in which women's and men's experiences are influenced by race and class. Feminist scholarship has deconstructed and challenged traditional views of family life and explored family as a site of struggle and domination in the following ways:

> (1) normative superiority of the traditional nuclear family and (2) the ideology of family life as the center of loving relations. Beginning with women's experiences, feminist scholars have both problematized and enriched the concept of family. In exploding the myth of the universal, emotionally satisfying nuclear family, by making visible the existence and strength of very diverse family forms, socialist feminists go beyond the notion that biological reproduction is something all women want and in fact engage in and that, further, women's intermittent labor force participation alone causes poverty in old age.
>
> (Calasanti and Zajicek 1993: 124)

The nuclear family is not the key to understanding family experiences of older adults since there is diversity within families. Stoller and Gibson (2004: 281–3) point out that some older adults did not marry or have children, some women have found their experiences as full-time housewife and mother to be more nega-tive than the idealized view, some women have engaged in paid employment at the same time as rearing young children, African American families have expe-rienced strict gender role division of household responsibilities less frequently than White families, complex networks of female kin exist in many families, and the idealized family image ignores lesbian women and gay men by assuming that the family consists of a heterosexual couple. Calasanti and Zajicek (1993: 125) note that in spite of struggle and domination within families, "relations may be more cooperative than conflictual among racial/ethnic groups as the family becomes a site of resistance to oppression in the broader society."

Sociological understanding of experiences of older adults in retirement has also been increased by socialist feminist scholars who have addressed the gendered welfare system as a component of state policies. The assumption that women are dependent on men has been reinforced through inequities in Social Security in the United States benefits based on the assumption that women would not be working outside of the home (Calasanti and Zajicek 1993). From the perspective of intersectionality, it is important to understand effects of both race and gender on retirement. African American women had relatively consistent participation in the labor force during the twentieth century, but the relatively low wages of many African American women compared to White women resulted in their position as a group with one of the lowest retirement incomes (Calasanti and Slevin 2001: 107).

According to Calasanti and Zajicek (1993: 125), analyses that are especially useful for developing understanding of policies perpetuating gender inequalities are those that "view the state in a historical, dynamic manner, acknowledge the role of contradictory social struggles, and argue that the challenge to state-based patriarchal dominance depends on women's political agency." Calasanti and Slevin (2001: 109) explain that there are two primary reasons for the continuing gender differential in salaries of men and women in the U.S. These are: (1) the need of many women to consider family obligations in their decisions regarding jobs and work schedules; and (2) obstacles that some women who want to work full time encounter in obtaining high-status jobs and promotions because of employers' assumptions that home responsibilities will distract them from their employment responsibilities. These experiences also contribute to more women than men entering retirement with financial disadvantage. Mandel and Shalev's (2009) assessment of the impact of the welfare state on cross-national variation in the gender wage gap indicates that the state influences gender inequality in labor market attainments through its influence on women's class positions and regulation of class inequality.

Feminist political economy of aging theories

The feminist political economy of aging perspective aims to understand how vulnerability and dependency of women throughout their lives is rendered by dominant social institutions, particularly economic and political systems.

According to political economy of aging theorist Carroll Estes (2006: 81), this approach includes analysis of:

> ...how state policies differ, individualize, and commodify the problems of aging (e.g., as individual problems and personal private responsibility for the purchase of services sold for profit) (Estes, 1979), and how these processes are ideologically and practically consistent with state roles and activities that advance the interests of capital accumulation and the legitimation of patriarchal and capitalist social relations.

Estes (2006: 81–2) states that four premises are fundamental to this approach. First, women's lives are socially constructed throughout life, particularly in social roles and responsibilities in relationships between men and women and in the institutional configurations of family state, and the labor market. Second, lived experiences and problems of women are primarily socially constructed rather than largely the result of individual behavior and decisions. Women are constrained by gender regimes in the capitalist state, the market, and the family. The third premise asserts that women's disadvantages are cumulative throughout life, and the fourth premise is that "the feminization of poverty is inextricably linked to the complex and interlocking oppressions of race, ethnicity, class, sexuality, and nation that produce the marginalization of older women."

The feminist political economy of aging perspective on aging and old age policy views study of the state as fundamental to understanding opportunities of older women because the state has the power to "(a) allocate and distribute scarce resources to ensure the survival and growth of the economy, (b) mediate between the different needs and demands across different social groups (gender, race, ethnicity, class, and age), and (c) ameliorate social conditions that could threaten the existing order" (Estes 2006: 84). Women's statuses as citizens, clients of state welfare services (especially likely with increasing dependency with age), and public employees connect them to the state. The institutions of family, state, and market mediate between women and society (Estes 2006).

According to theorists Beverly Ovrebo and Meredith Minkler (1993), objective realities of women's lives are related to structural inequalities connected to intersecting trajectories of gender, class, sexual orientation, and race. They explored the role of gender in aging with a dual focus, addressing gender's political significance relative to structural constraints and its potential to illuminate existential questions. They chose to explore gender and aging from a perspective outside of the more usual social science or existential and humanistic frameworks and focus on the tradition exemplified by philosopher Simone de Beauvoir. In *The Coming of Age* (1970) and *The Second Sex* (1972), de Beauvoir focused on objective data as well as subjective experience to explore intersections between political economy and meaning (Ovrebo and Minkler 1993: 290). According to Ovrebo and Minkler (1993: 290–1):

> Beauvoir (1970) saw social stratification in Western societies as based on utilitarian ethos, wherein humans are valued contingently, in terms of their

worth as producers and consumers. In contrast, a social justice perspective presupposes the valuation of humans unconditionally, what Frankl (1990) terms a person's 'dignity' and Kant (1789), the view of human beings as 'sacred ends.' The quest for meaning, for a life with purpose, begins with experiencing one's dignity as a human being. How is aging with dignity achieved in a society that values people in terms of their conditional and instrumental value? And how do those who are systematically and structurally devalued because of their gender, age, class, race, and/or sexual identify [sic] find and make meaning of their old age?

Consistent with political economy perspectives, Brown (1995) developed a theory of "state masculinism" and considers this to have the following characteristics:

1. *Juridical-legislative* – the formal and constitutional rights in which civil society is seen as a masculine right in relation to the natural and prepolitical place of women and the family.
2. *Capitalist* – the defined property rights and the possibilities for active involvement in wealth accumulation.
3. *Prerogative* – the [state's] legitimate monopoly of force and violence.
4. *Bureaucratic* – expressed through the institution of the state and its discourse, as discipline, presented as a neutral means of power. This makes it especially potent in shaping the lives of female clients of the state.

(Estes 2006: 85)

Estes (2006: 85) considers state masculinism to have the following policy implications for the lives of older women:

Reflecting the juridical-legislative state role, the caregiving role of women is assumed as the natural and prepolitical place of females. Under the state's role *vis-à-vis* capitalism, property rights and the ability to accumulate wealth are limited by the impaired ability of women to actively access paid employment as a result of their substantial caregiving responsibilities and sexism in the workplace (Ferree & Hall, 1996; Orloff, 1993). In the state's prerogative role, violence, hate crimes against women, and state control of reproductive options each profoundly shape women's opportunities for participation and livelihood in the society. In the state's bureaucratic role, older women, as clients of welfare and other state assistance programs, must deal with demeaning and unequal power relationships with state agents of social control.

A feminist perspective on masculinities and aging

Feminist theories and research about men's lives result from understanding that both femininity and masculinity need to be viewed as social constructs that change over time within cultural and national contexts. Feminist theorists also emphasize the importance of understanding gendered power relationships.

Robert Meadows and Kate Davidson's (2006) analysis of findings from a study of older men reflects the feminist trend toward theorizing beyond a simplistic view of men as a privileged sex class and recognizing that other statuses need to be taken into account. They assert that attention to the lives of old men provides insights that have the potential to inform, challenge, and change feminist theory, practice, and research and that age relations "present critical axes of inequality" through which old men are subordinated, especially in relation to younger men (2006: 295).

Gerontological theorizing about older men has resulted in varied conceptualizations. Some gerontologists believe that old men are emasculated by aging while others believe that aging men adapt to a new, similar, dominant ideological experience of masculinity (Thompson 1994). According to Connell (1995), multiple masculinities coexist and compete for dominance in any time and place, and the most desired, "hegemonic masculinity," tends to be dominant (Connell 2000: 10). Kimmel and Messner (2004) believe that at times male privilege is muted when physical abilities, as well as race, social class, sexual orientation, and immigration and national status are considered (Baca Zinn et al. 2007: 151).

Meadows and Davidson's (2006: 296), description of hegemonic masculinity provides insights about the need for feminist explorations of masculinity and aging:

> Hegemonic masculinity refers to those behaviors and practices that embody the 'currently accepted answer to the problem of the legitimacy of patriarchy,' which makes a successful claim to authority and which guarantee the dominant position of men over women (and other men) (Connell 1995: 77; Coates 2003). Within contemporary Western societies, the dominant, hegemonic ideology is said to prioritize such traits as physical strength, virility, wealth, self-control, and aggression (Calasanti 2004). It is also said to prioritize youth (Whitehead 2002). As men age, their withdrawal from the occupational breadwinner role, their possible loss of sexual potency, their diminishing physical strength, and the onset of illness can all weaken their relationship with this dominant ideology (Arber, Davidson, &Ginn 2003).
>
> In a circular and somewhat paradoxical manner, the study of old men can uncover 'the young and middle-aged biases that inhere in typical notions of masculinity' (Calasanti & King 2005: 19) precisely because these typical notions are age dependent and so are no longer available to many old men. In essence, old men are *absent* from a masculinized space and, as a result, are often awarded the status of 'other.'

Meadows and Davidson (2006: 296–7) analyzed narratives from the perspective of feminist theory that were obtained in research interviews with 85 Caucasian men over the age of 65 in the United Kingdom. They regard the older men in the study to be absent from hegemonic space because of their ages and assert that this enabled the respondents to provide insights into hegemonic forms of masculinity. Changes in the men's production and power relations and emotional attachments also enabled them to provide insights into coping strategies that they used to respond to loss of the hegemonic space.

In their analysis of the data, Meadows and Davidson (2006: 296):

> ...draw on Renold's suggestions that notions of otherness are reinforced not only through being absent from a masculinized space but also through *inhabiting* spaces associated with 'emphasized femininity' (2004: 252). These spaces are defined around compliance with subordination and orientated to supporting the desires and wishes of men (Connell 1987: 183). Providing care, for example, is a labor reserved principally for women (Calasanti 2004) and, as a result, tends to be seen as a feminine space. As men age, they not only become absent from youth-oriented hegemonic forms of masculinity but also increase their chances of inhabiting feminine space. Those who occupy these feminine spaces also invoke strategies in an attempt to remain approximated to hegemonic forms.

Changes identified by the men included loss of the roles that they possessed as members of the dominant group of younger males. These included their roles as provider (breadwinner), a role in the arena of production relations that they mourned. They also experienced changes in power and sexual prowess that Meadows and Davidson interpret as changes linked with emotional relations. The respondents' identification of these losses reflected the importance of these capabilities to the men and their significance in relation to hegemonic masculinity (Meadows and Davidson 2006: 298).

Production relations include "structuring of production, consumption, and distribution (Connell 1987: 103) and involve the gendered allocation of tasks and the nature and organization of this work" (Meadows and Davidson 2006: 299). The changing nature of gendered distribution of work was mourned by some of the respondents, including Kevin:

> Kevin, who was 'pretty senior' in his business, noted that his wife did her part by being 'absolutely super at entertaining' and made a 'good wife and mother.' Kevin continued to explain that since his wife had died, he had missed the 'normal' division of labor. 'I now have to undertake considerable domesticity, which I hate. I miss the normal marital relationship.'
>
> (Meadows and Davidson 2006: 299)

Some of the men, including Angus, described problematic changes in production relations that were related to loss of physical abilities: "'For many years I've told myself, in terms of physical ability, that I would still do everything that I did when I was twenty. Now in the last five years I've had to accept that, you know, that's a dream...and it's tough'" (Meadows and Davidson 2006: 300). Respondents' descriptions of loss of bodily performance were synonymous with descriptions of loss of manliness and illustrated changes in power relations as well as production relations (Meadows and Davidson 2006).

Themes of dominance and subordination with regard to gender and age appeared in the respondents' narratives and reflected changes in the men's experiences as they became older:

> Within our study the men's stories frequently turned to earlier demonstrations of power over women and children. Clive offered a particularly lengthy discussion of how, despite his son's insistence that his financial affairs had nothing to do with him, he took control of his son's bank account and 'made him' pay into a savings bond. Similarly, the data are replete with stories of men putting their foot down with their wives and knowing best what would be good for them....
>
> The prevalence of these stories was again amplified by the fact that this power was now receding for many of the men....Furthermore, for some men 'a lack of respect from the young' manifested itself into fear of walking into certain parts of their towns and fear of encountering intimidation and verbal abuse.
>
> (Meadows and Davidson 2006: 300)

Old men become involved in struggles that may allow them to have an "alternative view of lived reality." Their loss of power has epistemological importance because aging provides opportunities for men to experience life as the "other" when they no longer belong to the "ruling gender," especially when their bodies deteriorate physically. This is consistent with the feminist view that a feminist standpoint is achieved when women engage in struggles that allow them to see an alternative reality of social life from perspectives shaped by oppression (Meadows and Davidson 2006: 301).

Meadows and Davidson (2006: 301) discuss changes in emotional relations of older men primarily in terms of "cathexis; that is, desire as emotional energy and the practices that shape this desire." The men in the study discussed their sexuality in terms of standards that they had for themselves in the past, and decline in sexual functioning could reinforce feelings of being old: "Clyde, for example, noted that a lack of sexual functioning created a sense of loss in his life, and he, arguably, was aware that this shifted him away from what he was supposed to be....He now had 'gaps' in his life, of which sex seemed to be a major component. Such gaps were a major theme throughout the data and represented men's realizations concerning where they should be in relation to hegemonic masculinity."

Nevertheless, Meadows and Davidson (2006: 302) found that the men resisted "otherness" that would distance them from their hegemonic expectations of themselves by finding strategies to approximate hegemony in production relations, power relations, and emotional relations. In production relations, they emphasized what they were still able to do and viewed aging as connected with physical decline rather than chronological age. Self-perception in power relations was maintained by a strategy of viewing oneself as better than others, which is consistent with social comparison literature in aging (Frisby 2004). A respondent in the study, Mike, said that his neighbor never goes outside and is not much older than Mike, and Meadows and Davidson (2006: 303) note that identifying "who is 'better' than is a value-laden exercise that reflects definitions of normalness and appropriate behavior. The process can engender a feeling of power within one group and feelings of powerlessness within others."

In the area of emotional relations, Meadows and Davidson (2006: 304) report that the men used a strategy of "exaggerated notions of heterosexual prowess and expulsion and disassociation of homosexuality (Renold 2004). For example, in a conversation about how he used to form friends with the opposite sex, Angus confirmed his heterosexual nature by stating the he likes 'the opposite sex...who doesn't?' and situated himself as normal by making jokes about homosexuality and those 'people who are different.'"

Similar strategies were used when the men occupied a "potentially feminized space. Emphasizing power, control, functional ability, and 'doing' remain favored strategies here" (Meadows and Davidson 2006: 304). Furthermore, intersectivity is also addressed in the interpretation of respondents' reactions to caregiving:

> A person's social location intersects with aging, adding further dimensions to the tensions that exist between aging and masculinities. On the more macroscale this can involve elements of an individual's race, gender, and class. On a microscale this can involve social situations, such as caregiving, that can locate the male within feminine spaces.
>
> For example, old men within our study attempted to combat the potentially negative image of caring in relation to their gender identity by defining it in functional, instrumental terms. As Kaye and Applegate suggest, the old male caregiving orientation is characterized by displays of 'rationality with feeling' (1994: 230). The employment-based identity transfers to the caregiving role (p. 228). Gary, for example, described how it was 'his job' to deal with his wife's death certificate, although his children had offered to attend to this, because he was her husband and lover for fifty-two years.

Respondent Darren described his preference to be his wife's caregiver rather than accept more assistance:

> We thought we'd get someone in to try to give it a try to wash her and dress her, but the ones they sent were tiny little women and of course Peg was rather tall, she was 5'10" or something, you see. And once or twice she used to call me to the bed, and of course they couldn't manage to lift her up, and with different girls each week, I thought, no, this is a waste of time, it's no good. So I said, 'No, don't worry, I'll do it myself'—so I did it myself. But we had a nurse come to bathe her on occasion, weekly or whatever it was. She did a tour of the district and she'd come here on the Friday morning or something like that, but the rest I did myself. Yes, I looked after her all the time. Just like doing another job, except indoors!
>
> (Meadows and Davidson 2006: 305)

Meadows and Davidson (2006) assert that men can continue to apply these strategies as they become older or they can adopt "alternative masculinities." When men do not have the resources to use the negotiation strategies mentioned above, they may discontinue their efforts to approximate hegemonic masculinity and attempt to develop alternatives. Others will continue to attempt hegemonic forms and believe that they are approximating hegemonic masculinity even when the efforts are not successful. In this study, respondents who engaged with alternative masculinities did so because they were a "physical wreck," according to Meadows and Davidson (2006: 307). They describe Earl's challenges:

> In relation to caring, Earl could not control his wife's decaying body as 'she always had bowel trouble.' In addition, lifting his wife 'fourteen times a day' became too much for his aging body to take and, despite having a home care assistant, no one was around to witness his caring during the majority of the day. He considered he had become 'invisible,' and his physical deterioration went unnoticed by those around him. The 'hard labor' of caring had taken a toll on his health, and even though he was only in his late sixties when she died, he felt unable to pursue activities such as playing bowls and joining social clubs, which had been curtailed by his caring responsibilities. It is interesting that – and we don't wish to negate the love Earl obviously had for his wife – he was one of the few men who expressed feeling cheated because he had to care for his wife:
>
> I felt cheated. I felt cheated out of life. Because I was so lively, I was always full of fun when I was a youngster, always parties and I was always invited everywhere but I honestly after looking after her for thirty years, I feel as if I have been cheated.
>
> (Meadows and Davidson 2006: 308)

Meadows and Davidson (2006: 306–8) believe that feminisms are informed and challenged by focusing on the lives of old men. Through exploration of their lives, the defining attributes of hegemonic masculinities are illustrated, and narratives clarify that it is younger men who possess the society's ideal notions of manliness. Insights are also provided into coping strategies used to address tensions between masculine hegemony and aging. This exploration also offers emancipatory possibilities because everyone who lives to old age will experience loss of privileges because of aging regardless of the amount of privilege possessed earlier in life. The changes in men's "lived reality" have the potential for leading to a "men's anti-patriarchal standpoint" and greater understanding of women because of older men's increased sense of otherness due to their subjection to domination.

Summary

Feminist theory is a multidisciplinary area of critical theory with origins in civil rights and women's liberation movements that questioned the status quo during the last half of the twentieth century. Origins of feminist perspectives in sociology also include the influence of social constructionist and other postmodern approaches. Consistent with social constructionism, feminists deconstruct ideas, theories, and methods in order to understand their meanings and view knowledge as socially situated.

There have been several trends in development of feminist theory since the 1970s. Theories that emphasized differences between men and women were problematic because this led to overgeneralization and treatment of each category as a homogeneous category. Another development, the idea that femininity and subordination of women are social constructions, led to exploration of the social construction of masculinity and men's power. A stage of feminist thinking about gender grounded in diversity of experiences has existed since the mid-1980s, and this perspective views women and men in terms of their relationship to social structure and addresses relational aspects of gender. Feminist theorists also point out that opportunities for human agency result from social stratification and that political theorizing leading to social changes is needed. Social changes by and on behalf of women are core incentives for feminist theorizing.

In feminist gerontology, opportunities and constraints related to gender and age are examined at individual, interactional, and institutional levels, and this includes attention to the aging of gendered selves, exploration of diverse cultural expectations for people of different ages and genders, and age and gender specific rules for distribution of resources and material items. Socialist feminist theories of aging are based on the belief that problematic life circumstances of older women have resulted from patriarchal and race-based definitions of the productive and reproductive activities acceptable for women and men and categorization of jobs have resulted in women's and men's different retirement experiences.

The feminist political economy of aging perspective endeavors to understand how vulnerability and dependency of women throughout their lives is rendered by dominant social institutions, particularly economic and political systems. This perspective on aging and old age policy views study of the state as fundamental to understanding opportunities of older women.

Feminist theories and research about men's lives result from understanding that both femininity and masculinity need to be viewed as social constructs that change over time within cultural and national contexts. Feminist theorists also emphasize the importance of understanding gendered power relationships. Robert Meadows and Kate Davidson's study of hegemonic masculinity in older men addresses diversity of experiences in aging and provides insights into axes of inequality through which older men are subordinated on the basis of age.

6   Life course gerontology

Key concepts

1. Sociologist Glen H. Elder, Jr.'s, life course analysis of longitudinal data about the lives of individuals who grew up in the U.S. during the Great Depression in the 1930s contributed to development of life course theory by identifying the need for new theories and research focusing on historical influences on family, education, and work roles.

2. Additional impetus for developing the life course perspective came from the field of social history, with its emphasis on the importance of obtaining knowledge about ordinary people's experiences from people themselves rather than telling the story from the perspectives of wealthy and powerful individuals.

3. Life course theory also has roots in traditional theories of developmental psychology but differs especially because of attention in the life course perspective to ways that social location, historical time, and culture affect people's experiences.

4. Major themes in the life course perspective are interplay of human lives and historical time, timing of lives, linked or interdependent lives, human agency in making choices, diversity in life course trajectories, and developmental risk and protection.

5. Elder developed the life course paradigm principles of historical time and place, timing in lives, linked lives, and human agency based on his analysis of "Children of the Great Depression."

6. The life course perspective requires consideration of experiences throughout a person's life, but a gerontological life course perspective focuses primarily on understanding the effects of life course experiences on older adults.

7. Sociologist Matilda White Riley's theories of aging, social change, and the life course that were developed with colleagues John Riley, Jr., and Anne Foner address the relationship between social change and the behavior of individuals within social institutions.

8. Riley considered age to be a structural aspect of any changing group or society, and individuals and social changes continuously influence each other as people age.

9. Riley's aging and society paradigm is useful for visualization of the reciprocal relationship between macro-level social changes and individuals as micro-level systems.

10. According to Riley, structural lag exists when lives have been changing but society's compensatory structural changes lag far behind, producing strains for individuals and society as a whole.

11. Eleanor Campbell Stoller and Rose Gibson introduced an approach to the life course perspective that provides a broad perspective for understanding diversity in the aging process by including elements of personal biography, sociocultural factors, and sociohistorical periods.

12. Stoller and Gibson view gender, race, ethnicity, and social class as social constructs that are manifested in labels assigned to individuals within multiple hierarchical social structures and affect opportunities throughout the life course.

13. Ferraro, Shippee, and Schafer's integration of cumulative advantage/disadvantage theory focuses on population and cohort differentiation from a life course perspective that enables them to address how cumulative inequality develops.

Introduction

Chapter 6 provides an introduction to life course perspectives, including major life course concepts, followed by discussion of life course gerontology. Glen H. Elder, Jr.'s, seminal life course analysis about people who experienced childhood in the United States during the economic depression of the 1930s and the life course theoretical concepts derived from this analysis are explained. Life course concepts in social gerontology are discussed, especially concepts in Matilda White Riley's sociology of age which are also used for analysis of findings in Patricia Kolb's study of nursing home placement of African American, Afro-Caribbean, Latino, and White Jewish older adults in the United States. Eleanor Palo Stoller and Rose Campbell Gibson's life course perspective that addresses the relevance of gender, race, ethnicity, and social class for understanding the effects of lifelong experiences on later adulthood add to understanding of diversity. This is used for analysis of experiences of a Puerto Rican family living in New York City during the 1930s and 1940s. The chapter concludes with analysis of cumulative inequality theory vis-à-vis cumulative advantage/disadvantage theory and discussion of future development of life course theories.

Foundations of life course theory

Life course theory includes perspectives introduced during the twentieth century in the work of sociologists, psychologists, anthropologists, social historians, and demographers. Sociologist Glen H. Elder, Jr.'s (1999) life course analysis of longitudinal data about experiences of individuals who grew up in the U.S. during the Great Depression in the 1930s was influential in development of this perspective during the 1960s and 1970s. His contributions to life course theory continue to influence life course research. Elder's analysis was based on data from longitudinal studies of children in research conducted by social scientists at the University of California, Berkeley, beginning in 1932, and he focused primarily on a group of children born in Oakland, California, in 1920–1. Elder identified the need for new theories and research focusing on historical influences on family, education, and work roles.

Additional influences on development of the life course perspective came from the field of social history, with its emphasis on the importance of obtaining knowledge about ordinary people's experiences from people themselves rather than telling the story from the perspectives of wealthy and powerful individuals. A social historian, Tamara Hareven (1978, 1996, 2000), was instrumental in developing a focus on history of the family through examination of change and adaptation in families under different historical conditions. Life course theory also has roots in traditional theories of developmental psychology but differs especially because of life course perspective's attention to ways that historical time, social location, and culture affect people's experiences (Hutchison 2011: 10–11).

Glen H. Elder, Jr.'s, life course analysis: Children of the Great Depression

Elder began this life course study after his arrival at the University of California Institute of Human Development in Berkeley in 1962, and his book, *Children of the Great Depression: Social Change in Life Experience* (1999), provides detailed examination of his analysis and findings. In his analysis of archival data from the Oakland Growth Study that was initiated in 1931 at the Institute of Human Development by Herbert Stolz and Harold E. Jones in order to study aspects of pubertal transition of children born in 1920–1, Elder identified changes in individuals and families experiencing changing socioeconomic circumstances. In the Oakland Growth Study, data collection regarding the lives of 167 working-class, lower-middle-class, and middle-class fifth and sixth graders in five elementary schools in northeastern Oakland, California, began in 1932, and their physical, intellectual, and social development was studied from 1932 to 1939. Additional data about 145 members of the sample was collected in 1953–4, 1957–8, and 1964. They experienced life transitions as members of a cohort that lived through the economic depression of the 1930s as children, participated in military service during World War II, gave birth to the baby boom generation, and experienced parenthood during the generation gap in the 1960s. During World War II, most of the males in the study served an average of three years in the military, marriage took place for most of the women and men during the war, couples' first child was born during the period of relative affluence after the war, and in the postwar years the females were occupied with child rearing. Many of their baby boom children enrolled in college during the 1960s.

Elder's analysis of longitudinal data about this study group focused on the "life course from late adolescence to middle age; an assessment of the impact of family hardship on aspects of the life course; and specification of conditions under which adult values are linked to economic deprivation" (Elder 1999: 151). Considering ways that social changes influenced their lives, Elder (1999: 151) observed that since employment had increased appreciably in the Oakland area and the United States was two years from entry into World War II by the time the study subjects graduated from high school in 1938–39, "By any standard, life opportunities were more favorable for the Oakland adolescents than for young Americans who came of age five or ten years earlier." New economic and educational opportunities became available for this group as a result of World War II. Elder also identified significant differences in the childhood of many of the Oakland subjects compared to that of their own children. Many of the Oakland subjects experienced deprivation during childhood; in contrast, many of their children experienced affluence when they were children.

Elder's comparison of experiences and historical circumstances of the participants in the Oakland Growth Study with the lives of research participants in the Berkeley Guidance Study who were born in 1928–9 was important in his development of life course theory. Participants in the Oakland Growth Study reached adolescence during the 1930s, but boys and girls in the Berkeley Guidance Study were younger dependent children throughout the Great Depression. Elder found that there were differences in the influence of economic changes on family members of the two groups of children, but families' adaptations to economic hardships were similar in the two cohorts. The boys in the Berkeley group were less hopeful, self-directed, or confident about the future than the girls in the Berkeley study and the children in the Oakland cohort. Furthermore, the greatest discontinuity between childhood and adult health was reflected in a range extending from impaired development to psychological competence for Berkeley men with deprived histories (Elder 1999: 317–18).

Based on his analysis, Elder (1999: 304–8) developed the following life course paradigm principles:

1. The principle of historical time and place: *"The life course of individuals is embedded in and shaped by the historical times and events they experience over a lifetime."*
2. The principle of timing in lives: *"The developmental impact of succession of life transitions or events is contingent on when they occur in a person's life."*
3. The principle of linked lives: *"Lives are lived interdependently, and social-historical influences are expressed through this network of shared relationships."*
4. The principle of human agency: *"Individuals construct their own life course through the choices and actions they take within the opportunities and constraints of history and social circumstances."*

Major life course concepts

Elder and other life course theorists have continued to focus on ways that people are influenced by chronological age, relationships, common life transitions, and social change throughout their lives. Consistent with Elder's earlier analyses, examination of the effects of these influences focuses on experiences of people within a cohort, defined as a "group of persons who were born during the same time period and who experience particular social changes within a given culture in the same sequence and at the same age" (Hutchison 2011: 11). The size of a cohort affects opportunities for education, work, and family life. For example, when the large "baby boom" cohort that was born in the United States between 1946 and 1964 entered the labor force, wages decreased and unemployment increased because of the greater number of people seeking employment. People studying responses to special circumstances within cohorts have identified strategies used to respond to these circumstances. It has been suggested that many "baby boomers" responded to their cohort's distinctive economic challenges with changes such as more mothers engaging in paid employment and couples delaying marriage and childbirth and having fewer children (Hutchison 2011).

Additional concepts that are commonly used in life course theorizing are transitions, trajectories, life events, and turning points. Transitions involve changes such as retirement that are considered a distinct departure from previous roles and statuses. Trajectories are long-term patterns of stability and change that involve multiple transitions but have continuity of direction. Because there are multiple spheres in people's lives, multiple intersecting trajectories such as family life and health trajectories exist. While trajectories tend to reflect continuity, they can involve discontinuity when life events become turning points. A life event is an occurrence involving a relatively abrupt change such as a wedding, illness, or death of a close family member that may produce effects that are serious and long lasting. A turning point is a major change in the life course trajectory. A life event such as an immigration experience can be a turning point for one person but not be for another (Hutchison 2011).

Development of life course gerontological theories

The life course perspective requires consideration of experiences throughout a person's life, but a gerontological life course perspective focuses primarily on understanding the effects of life course experiences on older adults. Sociologists have made essential contributions to this multidisciplinary perspective that includes micro- and macro-level analyses of individuals and populations and focuses on the entire life cycle, including deviations in trajectories. Researchers addressing later adulthood from this perspective attempt to explain:

1. the dynamic, contextual and processual nature of aging;
2. age-related transitions and life trajectories;
3. how ageing is related to and shaped by social contexts, cultural meanings and social structural location; and

4. how time, period and cohort shape the ageing process for individuals as well as for social groups (Bengtson and Allen, 1993; Elder, 1992; Elder and Johnson, 2002).

(Bengtson et al. 2005: 13–14)

Matilda White Riley: sociology of age

U.S. sociologist Matilda White Riley's theories of aging, social change, and the life course that were developed with principal collaborators John Riley, Jr. and Anne Foner address the relationship between social change and the behavior of individuals within the family and other social institutions. They have implications for understanding social change in many societies. Riley and her colleagues began to address age stratification in their work in the 1970s, and the intellectual roots of this perspective are in structural-functionalism, including work by Sorokin (1947), Mannheim (1928/1952), and Parsons (1942) (Bengtson et al. 2005).

Consistent with basic conceptualizations in the life course perspective, sociology of age views individuals as members of cohorts moving through their lifespan in different time periods, changing and being changed by societies through participation in social institutions such as the family. According to Riley, life stages are products of the interplay between aging, or development, and social change, and life stages are not fixed but vary with social change. Riley's approach includes: (1) aging throughout the life course; (2) societies and groups experiencing age stratification; and (3) successive cohorts providing linkages between aging individuals and age-stratified groups and societies. While individuals are engaged in living during different time periods, they create social change as they participate in social institutions throughout their lifespan. Riley considers age to be a structural aspect of any changing group or society, and individuals and social changes continuously influence each other as people age (Riley 1987).

According to Riley, life stages of individuals are the product of the interplay between aging, or development, and social change and do not result solely from biological, or ontogenetic, development (Riley 1986). There are variations in life stages that are related to social changes and changes in social structure over time, and Riley and Riley (1986: 55) proposed the following relevant principles:

1. In response to social change, people engage in new age-typical patterns and regularities of behavior (change in the way the aging process occurs);
2. As these behavior patterns become commonplace, they are defined as age-appropriate norms and rules, are reinforced by 'authorities,' and are thereby institutionalized in the role structure of society (change in the social structure);
3. In turn, these changes in age norms and social structures redirect or otherwise alter a panoply of age-related behaviors (further changes in the aging process); and so on.

Based on her observations that people and roles are interdependent, yet distinct, throughout changing historical periods, Riley developed her principle of cohort differences: "Because of the effect of changing structures on lives, members of different cohorts grow old in different ways." Furthermore, she believed that this principle led to "another interpretive fallacy: erroneously assuming that members of all cohorts will age in exactly the same fashion as members of our own cohort....the fallacy of *cohort-centrism*" (Riley 1994: 436, 38, 40).

Aging and society paradigm

Sociology of age "provides an analytical framework for understanding the interplay between human lives and changing social structures" (Riley 1987: 1). Riley's aging and society paradigm is a component of this analytical framework that enables us to visualize the reciprocal relationship between macro-level social changes and individuals as micro-level systems. It allows us to visualize the transactional relationship between individuals throughout their lifespan, a lifespan in which life expectancy is increasing and structural changes are occurring within the institution of the family.

Riley's "aging and society paradigm" is illustrated in Figure 6.1 (Riley 1994: 441). This paradigm includes a diachronic view that is a multidimensional view linking past, present, and future, and links the dynamisms of changes in lives and in structures. It incorporates a synchronic view that is a cross-sectional "snapshot" or "slice" of age strata. The perpendicular lines indicate families or other social structures that influence lives of individuals as they exist in different historical times (Riley 1994: 436, 40, 48).

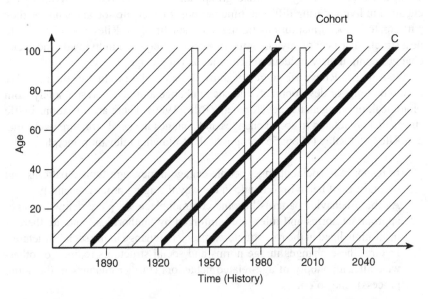

Figure 6.1 Diachronic View of the Paradigm: Changing Lives and Structural Change (Source: Riley 1994: 441). By permission of *The Gerontologist*/Oxford Journals.

The paradigm includes cohorts and identifies their flow through changing institutions such as the family, social welfare institutions, educational institutions, religious institutions, and employment institutions that affect the lives of individuals. When these institutions are studied over time, knowledge of structural changes such as changing life expectancy, family structure, and roles and responsibilities of older adults can increase our understanding of the lives of individuals and groups.

Structural lag and structural integration

Riley and Riley (2004: 110) theorized that over several decades social structures that divide social roles of education, work, and retirement would be transformed so that greater age integration in society would occur. Age would have less power to determine when entry and exit from these social structures should occur and would not constrain expectations about performance. They based their predictions on the following proposition in sociology of age:

> ...in all known societies, human aging and changing social structures are distinct but interdependent dynamisms. Each influences the other (Riley, Johnson, & Foner, 1972). In modern societies, however, a perplexing problem has been developing for decades: the dynamism of aging has been outrunning the dynamism of structural change. This is the problem we call 'structural lag' (Riley, 1988). Essentially, there is an imbalance between the mounting numbers of long-lived people (the unprecedented transformation of aging) and the lack of productive and meaningful role opportunities – or places in the social structure – that can recognize, foster, and reward these capacities.

Elaborating on the development of structural lag, Riley and Riley (1986: 51) wrote:

> As longevity increases, the complex processes of aging from birth to death – biological, psychological, and social – are continuously being shaped by ongoing changes in structure and social roles. Meanwhile, as the life course is modified, pressures are generated for still further changes – in social structures, institutions, beliefs, norms, and values. In turn, these societal changes influence the nature of the life course. Thus, there is a continuing dialectic between the processes of aging and changing social structures. People who are growing up and growing old today differ from their predecessors in the markedly increased length of their lives, as well as in many other ways. Lives have been changing, but our society's compensatory structural changes lag far behind, producing strains both on individuals and society as a whole.

Addressing implications of twentieth century increases in life expectancy and increase in the number of years of retirement, Riley and Riley (2004) emphasized the robustness of the majority of older adults who are neither fully disabled nor institutionalized and are capable of contributing to society. They suggested that empty role structures for increasing numbers of "capable, motivated, and potentially productive older people" could not continue to exist and that "imminent changes…are underway that can help to offset the structural lag. These changes – though latent – are intrinsic to the continuing societal interplay between changing lives and continuing social structure" (Riley and Riley 1994: 111).

Riley and Riley (1994: 111–12) described the ideal type of "age-differentiated" structures that they viewed as reflective of the recent past and characterized by structural lag, and they described the contrasting ideal type of "age-integrated" structures in which age barriers are removed so that education, employment, and leisure opportunities are available to people of every age. Age-differentiated structures have been commonplace and divide social roles into educational roles for young people, work roles for middle-aged, and leisure or retirement for older people. Riley and Riley (1994: 111–12) doubted the continued viability of age-differentiated structures:

> Today, however, we believe that these age-based structures and norms can often be seen as vestigial remains of an earlier era when most people had died before their work was finished or their last child had left home. For example, age 65, established as the criterion for insurance eligibility in 19th century Germany, is still widely used under utterly changed contemporary conditions.
>
> Despite its failure to accommodate people's changing lives, this conventional age differentiation is continually reinforced. It has been appropriate for societies where paid work is the predominant role, and achievement (or material 'success') the predominant value. In particular, this age-differentiated type is bolstered by 'ageism,' the mistaken but stubborn belief in universal and inevitable decline because of aging: e.g., older workers, even those in their 50s, are erroneously believed to have inevitably lost their efficiency. Moreover, the familiar age-based divisions among education, work, and retirement offer many advantages: they provide orderliness as they have become 'institutionalized' in people's lives; they are a societal convenience; and they are typically accepted without question.

The contrasting ideal type, "age-integrated" structures, would provide role opportunities in education, work, and leisure to people of all ages, within the limits of biology:

> Ideally, such age-integrated structures would have revolutionary consequences. They would open to older people the full range of role choices. And, in changing the opportunities for older people, new opportunities would be unlocked for everyone. For the middle-aged, there would be reductions in the strains imposed by multiple roles – when work is combined with family, homemaking, and health care, as well as with leadership in politics,

religion, and community service. Ideally, too, such age-integrated structures would lead to the often proposed 'reconstruction of the life course,' providing options for people over their entire lives to intersperse periods of work with periods of education and of leisure. And for the society, these structures would broaden the economic base for support of that minority of older people who are frail and needy.

(Riley and Riley 1994: 112)

Riley and Riley (1994: 113) believed that there was already evidence of movement toward more age-integrated structures and that in the U.S. the greatest difficulties in reducing structural lag exist in "understanding how the changes occur and how particular *interventions* can operate to benefit, rather than damage, both individuals and society." Also, other forms of social integration and change are implicated in development of age-integrated structures, including new forms of institutional integration in which roles in work, leisure, and education intersect with roles in other social institutions to form new hybrids; gender integration into old age; and reassessment of values "as the norms [of achievement values and consumption aspirations] to which today's middle-aged people have been socialized encounter the exigencies of old age in an utterly changed future society" (Riley and Riley 1994: 114).

Sociology of age and analysis of admission to a skilled nursing (nursing home) facility

In the U.S., members of diverse ethnic and racial groups enter nursing homes for long-term care. Although Riley emphasized the significance of structural change in relation to relatively healthy older adults, her aging and society paradigm and concept of structural lag are also useful approaches for analysis of nursing home placement experiences. In Kolb's (2003) qualitative study of nursing home placement and adjustment of 75 African American, Afro-Caribbean, Latina/o residents, White Jewish residents, and their caregiving relatives and friends, interviews with the primary caregiving relatives and friends indicated that social changes created circumstances that resulted in the need for individuals in each group to find new ways to meet caregiving responsibilities that were traditionally assumed by relatives.

Nursing home placement is a deviation from traditional caregiving expectations of filial responsibility in many racial and ethnic groups. In the majority of the families in this study, nursing home placement deviated from caregiving behavior in previous cohorts. In 44 of the 75 families (59 percent), the resident did not have any relatives who had been admitted previously to a nursing home, and for 17 of the residents, only one relative had previously lived in a nursing home. The need for nursing home placement was identified as related to increased life expectancy, changes in women's roles and opportunities, socioeconomic challenges, and lack of viable alternatives for care that would ensure the safety of the frail older person.

As we have seen, Riley considered age to be an important social structural influence on people's lives. As a result of the demographic trend of increased life expectancy, more people are living long enough to need informal unpaid assistance from relatives and/or friends or assistance from paid formal service providers. In Kolb's study, the residents' ages at the time of nursing home admission reflected this trend toward increased life expectancy. They were between 58 and 99 years of age, with an average age of 80. Many of the relatives and friends who were the primary informal caregivers following admission were also older adults. They were between 22 and 91 years of age (Kolb 2003).

Marital statuses of the residents and their caregivers reflected changing trends in family structures in the United States. Twenty percent of the 75 caregivers were divorced, separated, or divorced and remarried. Twelve percent of the caregivers were widowed, and one was an unmarried individual living with a partner. Twenty-three percent were single, and 44 percent were married at the time of their interview (Kolb 2003).

The need for family members to be employed outside of the home was described by many of the participants as an impediment to providing the extensive care that was needed when older family members experienced severe health conditions. The effects of divorce on availability of females to be the traditional caregivers was reflected in employment rates since some women needed to be employed to support themselves following divorce. Fifty (67 percent), of all of the caregivers who were interviewed, were employed outside of their home at the time of the interview, with 39 (65 percent) of the 60 female caregivers employed at the time of their interview.

The participants discussed additional factors that contributed to the decision for nursing home placement. Multiple factors contributed to the need for placement for some residents, and for others a single acute episode of a medical condition precipitated placement. Additional challenges to families in meeting traditional caregiving expectations were related to the resident's history of migration or immigration that had resulted in a diminished number of relatives living near enough to provide needed assistance. Lack of accessible housing for mobility impaired individuals limited ability to remain at home; some residents had been on waiting lists for accessible public housing for many years. Space limitations in the homes of some family members prevented older adults from moving into a relative's home at the time that substantial assistance was needed although the older person and relative preferred this rather than nursing home placement. The cost of moving into more accessible and larger homes was prohibitive for many of the residents and their families (Kolb 2003).

All of the Latina/o residents and a majority of their caregivers were migrants from outside of the continental United States, and migration can result in a loss of housing options which provide more flexibility as well as the loss of the potential for assistance from the members of one's family (Drachman 1992). Many of the families had delayed nursing home placement for several years while their relative's health deteriorated, and the decision for nursing home admission was made when it became apparent that it was no longer safe for the older adult to live without 24-hour care and supervision. An African American daughter whose mother had been admitted to the nursing home two years prior to the research interview explained her family's experiences that resulted in the placement decision:

> She had a couple of falls at home, and we didn't know what was happening. Then, all of a sudden her level of consciousness just totally changed. We did not know what was happening with her, and we hired someone to come in and stay with her because she was really confused, and she was changing rapidly. A physician I know offered to come to her house and see her. He thought she needed to be admitted to the hospital, and he came to her home and said we definitely need to admit her. Before her level of consciousness changed, she said she didn't want to go to the emergency room, so this doctor admitted her to the hospital and she didn't need to go to the emergency room. She was seen by a neurologist who said that she had a hematoma, partly old, partly new. It had filled up so much of the cranial space by now that we were seeing the symptoms, but it could have been happening for years. They had to go in and evacuate, and once they evacuated it, she lost a lot of her functioning and we just knew that she could never go back home and live alone again. In fact, before this happened, we actually wanted her to have a home health aide and she totally refused. I mean she was 92... like ma!
>
> (Kolb 2003: 7)

Structural lag and nursing home placement decisions

Since Riley's (1994) paradigm shown in Figure 6.1 provides a valuable theoretical framework for explaining the reciprocal and lifelong relationship between allocation of roles for people at different ages and socialization for roles such as elder care, it is a useful tool for explaining cohort and sub-cohort changes in practices in family caregiving for older adults and the potential for structural lag. Use of the paradigm provides clarification about the relationship between structural changes such as increased life expectancy and changes in women's roles and ensuing changes in familial practices for provision of elder care. Riley's paradigm, with its timeline across the bottom of the diagram, represents the flow of cohorts in which familial roles may change over time. Her diachronic, historical, view of changing lives and structural change is useful for explaining cohort changes over time in decision-making regarding assistance for older adults in need of help. In Riley's synchronic view, it is accepted that there are changes over time in the allocation of people at particular ages to roles available to them and in the socialization of new 'recruits,' members of society, to meet role expectations for responsibilities such as care of older relatives. Structural lag in resources to meet caregiving needs may occur.

Riley's concept of structural lag facilitates consideration of the fact that many of the residents and their families preferred continued residence in the community, but placement occurred because of lack of adequate alternatives to institutionalization. Family members believed that there were no viable alternatives to institutionalization at the time of their relative's admission to the nursing home. Most of the residents had received assistance from family and/or friends and some had received assistance from formal home care agencies prior to nursing home admission but reached a time when care available at home was inadequate to meet their needs. Several of the residents needed home care for 24 hours a day, seven days per week, but were unable to obtain adequate publicly funded care and could not afford the high cost of home care paid for privately in order to remain outside of a nursing home.

Because of structural changes, the realities for contemporary cohorts of older persons, their relatives, and friends who made decisions about the care of older persons were different from the circumstances for previous cohorts. Admission of a relative to a nursing home deviated from caregiving behavior in previous cohorts in the majority of the families, and for many of the caregivers this was an extremely difficult decision. In 54 families, including families from each ethnic and racial category, no relatives had been admitted to a nursing home previously, and 17 residents had only one relative who had experienced long-term care in a nursing home. A cohort change in fulfilling caregiving roles in these families took place when a relative moved into the nursing home rather than continuing to live in the community. Admission to the nursing home occurred because of lack of informal and formal care providers to provide adequate community care and lack of viable community housing options.

A view of the aging experiences of individuals from the perspective of social change increases understanding of the variables to consider for effective service delivery, planning, and research. Although nursing home placement may continue to be antithetical to the culturally valued expectations of care for older relatives in many ethnic and racial groups, it nevertheless has become a reality for some group members. Findings from this study indicate a relationship between the social changes of increased life expectancy and the reduced availability of women as the traditional caregivers in some families to perform caregiving responsibilities for older relatives and the decision to place a relative in the nursing home. However, since the reality is that there have also been women in earlier cohorts who were employed, especially women belonging to ethnic and racial minority groups and women who were poor, multiple variables influencing changing elder care practices need to be considered and their interrelatedness understood. Thus, the changing nature of the tasks in women's employment and the changing nature of the demands on caregivers as their relatives and friends live longer are also important variables to be explored.

The study indicated that the emotional consequences of this nontraditional behavior within the context of traditional expectations can be profound for older persons in need of care and for their relatives and friends. When nursing home placement is considered, older people in need of assistance and their relatives and friends need information and support. Particularly when placement is being considered by persons belonging to ethnic and racial communities in which there is little or no prior experience with this and in which placement is not condoned, older people and their relatives and friends may need assistance from social workers and other staff in community agencies, hospitals, and nursing homes in order to make informed decisions. From a planning perspective, it is important to identify and address any gaps in resources that are constraints related to structural lag. Riley's (1994: 1216) affirmation that cohort differences require development of present and future interventions to improve lives is consistent with the implications of Kolb's research that unmet needs due to structural lag need to be addressed by developing more alternatives to nursing home placement.

Eleanor Palo Stoller and Rose Campbell Gibson: gender, race, ethnicity, and social class and life course theory

Stoller and Gibson (2000) introduced their approach to the life course perspective to provide a broader perspective for understanding diversity in the aging process by including elements of personal biography, sociocultural factors, and sociohistorical periods. They view gender, race, ethnicity, and social class as social constructs that are manifested in labels assigned to individuals within multiple hierarchical social structures, and their effects on opportunities throughout the life course and influence on aging experiences are important to consider. Listening to diverse voices provides a broader perspective by offering new lenses to view diverse social worlds.

The main premises of Stoller and Gibson's (2000: 19) life course perspective as an inclusive approach for understanding aging are:

1.   The aging process is affected by individuals' personal attributes, their particular life events, and how they adapt to these events.
2.   Sociohistorical times shape opportunity structures differently for individuals with specific personal characteristics, such as being in a subordinate position in a social hierarchy. Thus, people's life events, adaptive resources, and aging experiences differ.
3.   Membership in a specific birth cohort (i.e., being born in a particular time period) shapes the aging experience. Within cohorts, however, the experience of aging differs depending on one's position in systems of inequality based on gender, race, ethnicity, or class.
4.   Sociohistorical periods shape the aging experiences of cohorts. These historical times, however, have different impacts on the experiences of disadvantaged and privileged members of the same cohort.

Stoller and Gibson (2000) propose that there are patterns in experiences of groups within the older population that reflect cultural blueprints and social structural arrangements that structure different worlds in aging. Accumulation of disadvantages creates greater risks for negative outcomes, and these are circumstances that result in multiple jeopardy. Accumulation of privileges results from unearned ascribed advantages leading to greater quantities of accumulated resources, relationships, and definitions of social reality in old age. They point out that privileged and disadvantaged are complex terms because an individual can be privileged in some hierarchical areas and disadvantaged in others. Furthermore, while the multiple jeopardy approach to understanding inequality in old age tends to emphasize negative outcomes resulting from disadvantages, Stoller and Gibson also indicate that strengths can develop from living in disadvantaged positions.

Stoller and Gibson (2000) also address the importance of attention to sub-cohorts in order to understand inequalities related to differences in life events and adaptive resources of cohort members. In *Worlds of Difference: Inequality in the Aging Experience* (2000), they address the experiences of people belonging to various ethnic and racial groups within specific cohorts and provide the example of experiences of adults and children in Piri Thomas's Puerto Rican family in New York City before and during World War II. They provide excerpts from Thomas's novel, *Down These Mean Streets*, to illustrate the adaptive resources of disadvantaged members of systems of inequality and the economic function of the war for his family in El Barrio (Spanish Harlem).

Thomas (in Stoller and Gibson 2000: 44–6) wrote about his family's experiences during winter in their cold apartment:

> We drank hot cocoa and talked about summertime. Momma talked about Puerto Rico and how great it was, and how she'd like to go back one day, and how it was warm all the time there and no matter how poor you were over there, you could always live on green bananas, *bacalao* [codfish], and rice and beans. *"Dios mio,"* [My God] she said, "I don't think I'll ever see my island again."...
>
> The door opened and put an end to the kitchen yak. It was Poppa coming home from work. He came into the kitchen and brought all the cold with him...
>
> And Poppa looking at Momma and us, thinking how did he get trapped and why did he love us so much that he dug in damn snow to give us a piece of chance? And why couldn't he make it from home, maybe, and just keep running?
>
> And Miriam, James, Jose, Paulie, and me just looking and thinking about snowballs and Puerto Rico and summertime in the street and whether we were gonna live like this forever and not know enough to be sorry for ourselves....
>
> The next day the Japanese bombed Pearl Harbor.
>
> "My God," said Poppa. "We're at war."
>
> *"Dios mio,"* [My God] said Momma.
>
> I turned to James. "Can you beat that," I said.
>
> "Yeah," he nodded. "What's it mean?"
>
> "What's it mean" I said. "You gotta ask, dopey? It means a rumble is on, and a big one, too."

I wondered if the war was gonna make things worse than they were for us. But it didn't. A few weeks later Poppa got a job in an airplane factory. "How about that?" he said happily. "Things are looking up for us."

We can relate experiences of Thomas's depression-era family to Elder's (1999: 304–8) life course paradigm principles based on his analysis of "children of the great depression." Experiences of Thomas's family members with their differences in age, gender, roles, and cultural histories within one family provide additional examples of the principle of historical time and place in which each person's life course is embedded in and shaped by historical times, events, and locations. Furthermore, their experiences are insightfully described as unique for each family member, and as adults and children in New York City during the economic depression and the beginning of World War II, shared circumstances could still contribute to different life trajectories for each individual that reflect the principle of timing of events in the lives of individuals. Each child would be affected differently by the social and economic changes, and we can anticipate differential developmental impact of events such as their father's challenges with securing employment. The parents' ability to provide for their children and themselves and ensure a secure future for all is profoundly affected by the timing of crises and opportunities during the economic depression.

Elder's principle of linked lives is reflected in the effects of the Great Depression and entry of the U.S. into World War II on the experiences of family members and evident in the social and economic interdependence of Piri Thomas's family members. Effects of these sociohistorical circumstances on employment opportunities for Piri's father and related economic insecurity for the family could continue to affect the lives of the adults and the children and their relationships with each other after these historical events ended. The collective and individual coping mechanisms of family members had the potential for use in the future when they would be confronted with individual and family crises. Elder's principle of human agency is evident in the choices and actions that the family members used to cope with stressful life circumstances within the social and economic constraints and opportunities. Piri's father consistently availed himself of employment opportunities that were influenced by changing historical circumstances, regardless of the difficulties of the work, and he benefited from the support of his family. Stoller and Gibson (2000: 30) point out that in the period before World War II, Piri Thomas's family used their resources of family closeness and escape to memories of Puerto Rico to cope with stressful life events and poverty.

Cumulative inequality theory for research on aging and the life course

Stoller and Gibson addressed cumulative advantage/disadvantage theory, and Ferraro et al. (2009: 414–15) have also focused on the need to understand how early life events and status rankings are translated into outcomes in later life.

Ferraro et al. suggest that their perspective differs, however, because in developing their "cumulative inequality theory" they included elements subject to falsification and included "'sufficient formality' to differentiate closely related concepts," while also integrating life course theory into study of cumulative inequality and drawing heavily on the work of Dannefer (1987, 1988, 2003) and O'Rand (1996). Micro- and macro-sociological content is included in cumulative inequality theory in order to bridge both of these levels of analysis. Ferraro et al. (2009: 414) believe that questions such as "Do early events have impacts that are inexorable in their impact? Can early disadvantage be overcome? Are there compensatory mechanisms that can counter the general principle that 'the race is to the swift?' What role does human agency play in the process of cumulative disadvantage?" must be addressed in order for the concepts of cumulative disadvantage and cumulative advantage to be transformed into theory. There are five reasons why Ferraro et al. (2009: 414) regard cumulative inequality theory differently from cumulative advantage/disadvantage theory (CAD):

> First, the published record of CAD theory does not explicitly consider many elements that we deem essential to a theory for the study of cumulative inequality. One example that we articulate here is the intergenerational transmission of inequality. Thus, a slightly different phrase may help distinguish this articulation from the exemplary contributions of previous authors. Second, as is discussed, we think it is highly unlikely that cumulative advantage is the opposite of cumulative disadvantage. Whether the effect of disadvantage is parallel to that of advantage is an empirical question, but combining advantage and disadvantage in the name of the theory may be misleading. Third, cumulative inequality theory places the emphasis on system properties in generating inequality. Advantage and disadvantage are often seen as outcomes for given individuals, but the term *inequality* may help convey the importance of systemic properties in how individuals become stratified. Fourth, cumulative inequality theory gives explicit attention to *perceptions* of disadvantage rather than just the objective conditions of their situations, which has been the dominant approach in studies of accumulating disadvantage. Fifth, cumulative inequality is more concise than the phrase cumulative advantage/disadvantage.

Ferraro et al. (2009: 419) present cumulative inequality theory in five axioms with related propositions. The first axiom is "1. Social systems generate inequality – manifested over the life course via demographic and developmental processes." The related propositions identified below reflect important concepts for life course theory that are related to this axiom:

(a) Childhood conditions are important to adulthood, especially when differences in experience or status emerge early
(b) Reproduction is a fulcrum for defining life course trajectories and population aging

(c) Influenced by genes and environment, family lineage is critical to status differentiation early in the life course
(d) Cohorts provide the context for developing structuring risks and opportunities
(e) Consider inter- and intra-individual processes and use analytical techniques that explain variability on multiple levels or in multiple domains.

The second axiom is "2. Disadvantage increases exposure to risk but advantage increases exposure to opportunity." The related propositions are:

(a) Consequences of advantage may not be the inverse of disadvantage
(b) Inequality may diffuse across life domains (e.g., health and wealth)
(c) Trajectories are affected by the onset, duration, and magnitude of exposures.

The third axiom is "3. Life course trajectories are shaped by accumulation of risk, available resources, and human agency." The related propositions are:

(a) Human agency and resource mobilization may modify trajectories
(b) Turning points in the life course may alter the anticipated consequences of a chain of risk
(c) The dialectic of human agency and social structure is essential to cumulative inequality.

The fourth axiom is "4. The perception of life trajectories influences subsequent life trajectories." Related propositions are:

(a) Social comparisons shape trajectories
(b) Favorable life review is linked to self-efficacy
(c) Perceived life course timing influences psychosomatic processes.

The fifth axiom is "5. Cumulative inequality leads to premature mortality, perhaps giving the appearance of decreasing inequality in later life." Related propositions are:

(a) Cumulative inequality creates compositional change in a population
(b) Population truncation may give the appearance of decreasing inequality
(c) Test for selection effects
(d) Interpret results in light of event censoring and cohort inclusiveness.

Ferraro et al.'s (2009) integration of cumulative advantage/disadvantage theory that focuses on population and cohort differentiation with a life course perspective emphasizing the structure-agency dialectic enables theorists to develop their cumulative inequality theory that provides useful information for understanding how cumulative inequality develops.

Challenges for future development of life course theories: first principles and challenges to these in current life course analysis

Dale Dannefer and Jessica A. Kelley-Moore (2009: 407) assert that social inter-action and social structure should be considered first principles of life course analysis and that social structure has an important and irreducible role in organizing life course patterns. However, some life course theory and research neglects this focus, and Dannefer and Kelley-Moore (2009: 392) believe that despite advances in development of life course theory, six challenges for life course studies remain:

> (a) cohort analysis and the neglect of intracohort inequality, (b) confounding life course processes and change, (c) the need for renewed attention to inter-cohort variation, (d) time 1 encapsulation, (e) confounding the relation between age and time, and (f) expanding putative role of choice.

Elaborating on these challenges, Dannefer and Kelley-Moore (2009: 393) suggest that neglect of intracohort inequality occurred because "while the analytical tactic of comparing cohorts demonstrated the *importance* of context, it also allowed cohorts to stand as virtually *coterminous* with context so that the role of social forces operating within each cohort (e.g., regulating heterogeneity and homogeneity) received little attention." While intracohort stratification was identified as significant in Elder's (1974) work and the dynamics of diversity and inequality have received increased attention since the late 1980s, continued attention needs to be given to this area of life course theory and research (Dannefer and Kelley-Moore 2009: 393).

Dannefer and Kelley-Moore (2009) suggest that life course processes and change have been confounded by the tendency of life course theorists to give the variable of "cohort" a privileged conceptual status, and this "emphasis implies the salience of social change for understanding individual aging, and it invites the implicit assumption that social forces matter only in the case of social change." In reality, aging is socially constituted through fundamental processes of social interaction and allocation even when there are no large-scale changes in historical circumstances, and therefore under stable conditions aging should be treated as the master independent variable (Dannefer and Kelley-Moore 2009: 393–4)

Addressing challenges in theory and research regarding intercohort variations, Dannefer and Kelley-Moore (2009: 394) acknowledge the benefits of longitudinal studies that avoid the life course fallacy (Riley 1973) but believe that the commitment to longitudinal study of single age cohorts or adjacent cohorts is deficient in the area of age-period-cohort identification. They point out that study of a process within a single cohort and generalization of results to the larger population regardless of cohort confuses the theoretical maximum range of heterogeneity across cohorts with intracohort variability. This gives inadequate attention to embeddedness of individual lives in social structural and historical contexts.

The "time 1 encapsulation of social forces" problem refers to the fact that in much life course research social forces are "systematically considered at the initial observation period. When social-structural characteristics are considered only at Time 1, social structure at subsequent periods is unmeasured, and therefore treated as given" (Hagestad and Dannefer 2001: 7). This means that social forces affecting the individual's life in "time 1" are assumed to be characteristic of the individual later in life despite the fact that although "the original trajectory was set much earlier, social structure (and interaction with it) may lead to turning points, changes, or even reversals, and indeed the stability of the original trajectory depends in large part on a stable and predictable set of social relations and institutions" (Dannefer and Kelley-Moore 2009: 395).

The problem of confounding the relationship between age and time is related to the tendency to conceptualize and explain changes in health, social, and psychological functioning as a normative age pattern in a developmental framework. Dannefer and Kelley-Moore (2009: 395) point out that transitions, changes, and stability are often time-based phenomena and so it is important to be cautious about attributing change simply to aging.

The problem of "expanding putative role of choice" refers to the emphasis in the life course perspective on individual choice-making. Dannefer and Kelley-Moore (2009: 396) explain that in discussions about choice-making in the life course:

> What is almost always measured in such discussions is behavior, and it is simply *presumed* that behavior is based on choice. In such a usage of choice, the degree of constraints an individual feels and the differential levels of constraint that confront the individuals who have, for example, different health histories or who are differently located in opportunity structures are not analyzed. Nor is the degree to which perceptions and preferences are shaped by media-certified experts or by advertising.
>
> Without a systematic analysis of the life circumstances and subjective experiences that lie behind the observed behavior, an appealing and culturally familiar image of a volitional and more or less autonomous individual obscures the analytical problem of the constraints within which choices are made and the constitutive role of social interaction and social structure in constructing 'choice' in the first place.

Summary

Sociologist Glen H. Elder, Jr., has been a leader in the development of life course theory. His life course analysis of longitudinal data regarding the lives of individuals who grew up in the U.S. during the Great Depression in the 1930s contributed to identification of the need for new theories and research focusing on historical influences on family, education, and work roles. Based on his analysis, Elder theorized the life course paradigm principles of historical time and place, timing in lives, linked lives, and human agency. The fields of social history and traditional theories of developmental psychology were also influential in life course theory development.

Major themes in life course theory are interplay of human lives and historical time, timing of lives, linked or interdependent lives, human agency in making choices, diversity in life course trajectories, and developmental risk and protection. The life course perspective requires consideration of experiences throughout a person's life, but a gerontological life course perspective focuses primarily on understanding the effects of life course experiences on older adults. Sociologists Riley, Foner, and Riley had major roles in developing theories of aging, social change, and the life course that address the relationship between social change and the behavior of individuals within the family and other social institutions. Riley's aging and society paradigm enables us to visualize the reciprocal relationship between macro-level social changes and individuals as micro-level systems. Her concept of structural lag tells us that delays exist when lives have been changing, as with increased life expectancy, and structural changes lag far behind, resulting in individual and societal strains. The reality of lack of adequate resources for community living for some older adults who prefer to remain outside of nursing homes is an example of structural lag in an aging society.

Sociologists Stoller and Gibson introduced an approach to the life course perspective that provides a broad perspective for understanding diversity in aging experiences by including elements of personal biography, sociocultural factors, and sociohistorical periods. They view gender, race, ethnicity, and social class as social constructs that are reflected in labels applied to people and affect opportunities throughout the life course. They regard experiences of family members in Piri Thomas's *Down These Mean Streets* as illustrative of their perspective.

Ferraro, Shippee, and Schafer's integration of cumulative advantage/disadvantage theory focuses on population and cohort differentiation. Their life course perspective emphasizes a structure-agency dialectic that enables them to develop their cumulative inequality theory addressing how cumulative inequality develops.

7 Gerotranscendence

Key concepts

1. Swedish sociologist Lars Tornstam developed gerotranscendence theory as a meta-theoretical reformulation of disengagement theory and asserts that disengagement is a positive movement toward gerotranscendence that can be followed by increased life satisfaction.
2. According to Tornstam, gerotranscendence represents a positive shift in meta-perspective to a more cosmic and transcendent view compared to a materialistic and rational view.
3. According to gerotranscendence theory, the character, values, and meaning of old age are different from the attributes of the middle age years and there is continuous development in old age.
4. Movement toward gerotranscendence may involve changes in the cosmic dimension, the dimension of the self, and the dimension of social and personal relationships.
5. Tornstam believes that this transformative shift is less obvious in the U.S. than in cultures that recognize and support this shift in later life development, but it occurs in many societies and allows emergence of inner capacities that can compensate for and transcend physical and social losses.

Introduction

Chapter 7 describes the history of development of gerotranscendence theory by Swedish sociologist Lars Tornstam, followed by explanation of major concepts in Tornstam's conceptualization of gerotranscendence theory as a developmental theory of positive aging. Edmund Sherman's theory of contemplative aging that is consistent with gerotranscendence theory is described. Dimensions of gerotranscendence are described, and empirical support for gerotranscendence theory based on research in Denmark and Sweden is presented. Results of Fereshteh Ahmadi Lewin's cross-cultural analysis of findings from a study by Tornstam, Ahmadi Lewin, and L. Eugene Thomas of gerotranscendence and life satisfaction in Iranian older adults living in Sweden and Turks residing in Turkey are explained. Research about practice applications of gerotranscendence theory by Jannie Pevik Fasth and Barbro Wadensten in social work and nursing in Sweden is described. The chapter ends with Tornstam and Karin Hyse's case study of Mary, a gerotranscendent older woman in Sweden.

Foundations of gerotranscendence theory

Swedish sociologist Lars Tornstam (1992, 2005) developed gerotranscendence theory to address incongruities between empirical data and prevailing gerontological theories. This theory resulted from Tornstam's discomfort that much empirical data about aging did not match prevailing theories and that some theoretical attempts had been discarded. According to Tornstam (2005), overflow of functionalist presuppositions and values resulted in persistence of certain theoretical assumptions in gerontology, especially those reflecting a "misery perspective," and these were contradicted by empirical reality. Gerotranscendence theory addresses the need for a new meta-theoretical framework (Tornstam 2005: 12).

Tornstam (1989, 2005) developed this theory as a meta-theoretical reformulation of disengagement theory and asserts that disengagement is a positive movement toward gerotranscendence and can be followed by increased life satisfaction. Gerotranscendence theory is not a disguised form of disengagement theory, but an approach to understanding development in later life that differs from the dualism of disengagement versus activity (Hyse and Tornstam 2009, Sherman 2010). Gerotranscendence theory represents a positive shift in meta-perspective to a more cosmic and transcendent view compared to a materialistic and rational view. Understanding of this perspective requires shifting from a traditional Western positivist view of aging to phenomenological understanding of disengagement (Tornstam 1989, 2005). Although it has been suggested that Tornstam's development of gerotranscendence theory reflects an ambition to develop a "grand" theory, a meta-theory, of aging (Thorsen 1998), Tornstam (2011) states that gerotranscendence theory is not intended to be a meta-theory. The theory is meta- only in the sense of understanding something from a larger perspective (Tornstam 2011).

Gerotranscendence theory originated from Tornstam's eclectic knowledge of sociological, psychological, philosophical, spiritual, and anthropological perspectives, and fundamental influences were Cumming and Henry's (1961, 1963) formulation of disengagement theory and modifications or alternative explanations developed by gerontologists. Polish gerontologist Jerzy Piotrowski's views about disengagement theory and its counter theories influenced Tornstam's early thinking about disengagement theory, as well as Kuypers and Bengtson's (1973) concept of social breakdown syndrome that highlighted changes in thinking about disengagement. Additional influences included the work of Hakanson, Hochschild, Gutman, Jung, Fromm, Erikson, Peck and Chinen. Reports from acquaintances about direct work with older people influenced Tornstam's thinking about lived experiences of older adults and raised questions about existing theoretical perspectives. Tornstam (2011) considers gerotranscendence theory to be a grounded theory that has developed from the bottom up.

Disengagement theory and its relationship to
gerotranscendence theory

As indicated in the preceding section, Tornstam's (2005) formulation of gerotranscendence theory reflects his study and conversations about disengagement theory. The theorists who developed disengagement theory, Cumming and Henry, defined disengagement as "an inevitable process in which many of the relationships between a person and other members of society are severed, and those remaining are altered in quality" (1962: 211). Tornstam (2005) identifies three types of hypotheses in disengagement theory: (1) all societies push the aging person away, (2) the older person is intrinsically motivated to disengage from society socially and psychologically, (3) and the disengaged older adult continues to experience a high degree of contentedness, happiness, and life satisfaction. This suggests that if the disengagement process is violated and older adults are forced into activities, decreased satisfaction will ensue. This would be a result contrary to activity theory's premise that activity results in contentment and satisfaction.

Tornstam (2005) believes that many gerontologists reacted negatively to disengagement theory for two reasons. It was contrary to their humanistic orientation and their personal values that reflected a desire for later adulthood to be a continuation of their middle age lifestyle and because analysis of empirical data did not provide adequate support for the theory. According to Tornstam (1989, 2005), the hypothesis that Western societies reject old people is universally accepted, and this hypothesis is disengagement theory's sole indisputable support. He asserts that the second hypothesis has been dismissed by most gerontologists and that most, including himself, agree that if disengagement behavior exists it is not dependent on an intrinsic drive to disengage, but another influence. According to Tornstam, gerontologists have been especially interested in testing the third hypothesis (2005).

Tornstam (1989, 2005) identified Kuypers and Bengtson's (1973) theory of social breakdown syndrome, based on Zusman's (1966) social breakdown model of a negative social spiral resulting in social breakdown, as a perspective that reduced the disengagement pattern to social psychology and strongly influenced gerontological thinking about disengagement theory. Kuypers and Bengtson (1973) transferred Zusman's (1966) model of "the process by which the individual's social environment interacts with his/her self-perception in the production of a negative spiral – a social breakdown" to social gerontology and also presented a "model of social reconstruction, which described how the negative disengagement pattern could be broken... After this, the disengagement theory was referred to almost with disdain" (Tornstam 2005: 33, 34).

Subsequently, Tornstam (1989: 57–8) began to consider the possibility of congruence of activity theory and disengagement theory if they could be viewed within a different framework than the common positivist perspective. Influenced by Hakanson's (1981) discussions of meta-theoretical shifts, Hochschild's (1976) argument that phenomenological understanding is essential for understanding patterns of disengagement or engagement, and Gutman's (1976) movement toward a phenomenological description of the disengagement pattern in a cross-cultural study of Americans, Navajo Indians, low- and highland Maya Indians and Druzes, Tornstam proceeded toward development of a different kind of meta-theoretical paradigm. Tornstam's (1989, 2005) conceptualization was also influenced by findings from his study of experiences of loneliness of people between the ages of 15 and 80 in Sweden that indicated that degree of loneliness decreased for every consecutive age group despite the fact that participants experienced role and other losses. This suggested that some theoretical strengths might trail disengagement theory. Tornstam's (2005) study also found that there was a decrease for every consecutive age group in the positive effect of social interaction with other people as a remedy for loneliness.

Toward a meta-theoretical perspective for gerotranscendence theory

Tornstam (2005) identified a need to shift away from a positivistic paradigmatic framework in which there is an assumption of a common and shared definition of reality and the researcher defines the key concepts and what is considered normal. According to Tornstam, gerontology continues to bear the mark of traditional positivism because the borders of substantial parts of the prevailing research paradigm for gerontology essentially regard the elderly as research objects and the way that gerontologists define concepts and formulate theories is affected by presuppositions from society, especially values that emphasize productivity, effectiveness, and independence. Tornstam writes that theorists assume that old age implies continuity of values in middle age, but those values held in middle age may not be as important to people as they age. According to Tornstam, at times, theories such as role theory and activity theory have predominated in gerontology because of these points of departure. Therefore gerontologists have forced their own value-dependent theories on older adults, and deviations from these theoretical perspectives have been considered abnormal or pathological. Tornstam points out that the values imposed by theorists may not be the values of the older adults under consideration (2005).

As a developmental theory of positive aging, the gerotranscendence perspective stands in contrast to prevailing negative Western attitudes about older people (Sherman 2010, Tornstam 2005). Addressing negativity in Western attitudes toward older adults, Tornstam (2005: 12) writes: "White, Western, middle-class society has, since the Reformation, been characterized by an overwhelmingly strong performance orientation," and he asks "What happens to those in our society who do not live up to the ideal of productivity, effectiveness, and independence?" In his response, Tornstam cites Norwegian philosopher Harald Ofstad's (1972) work, indicating that we come to regard those who are considered unproductive, ineffective, and dependent, with contempt. Tornstam (2005: 12) continues: "To the extent that this applies to ourselves, we will do the same. We will regard ourselves with self-contempt. It is here that we find the basis for contempt towards unproductive, ineffective, and dependent old people, and a basis for the mismatch between theory and empirical findings." He notes that value patterns include various cultural sources, including old Hebrew tradition in which age and wisdom are highly regarded. Ofstad suggests that conflict between value patterns that generate contempt and those that generate respect tend to be resolved by hiding contempt or "changing it into something that allows it to be united with the respect for the elderly found in the Hebrew tradition" (Tornstam 2005: 12).

Tornstam's development of an alternative meta-theoretical paradigm was also influenced by his knowledge of Zen Buddhism and Jungian psychology. He considered the Zen Buddhist perspective that implies achievement of transcendence "in the sense that he lives in another, more boundary-free world compared with most of us from Western societies" (Tornstam 2005: 38). Tornstam (2005) noted that the meta-perspective of Zen Buddhists exists within Western philosophy in the psychological theories of C.G. Jung (1953) through Jung's description of a collective unconscious in which experiences of earlier generations and individuals are reflected in inherited structures in our minds and generations and individuals are unified through a collective unconscious that embraces structures and predispositions. Tornstam's initial conceptualization of gerotranscendence was also influenced by Jung's (1930) differentiation of meaning and tasks of midlife and old age. Jung suggested that in old age the task is to become acquainted with oneself and the collective unconscious, and earlier in life the task is to become acquainted with and socialized to society.

Gerotranscendence theory as a developmental theory of positive aging

Tornstam (2005) proposes that aging involves a process of increases in transcendence from young adulthood to old age. According to gerotranscendence theory, the character, values, and meaning of old age are different from the attributes of the middle age years, and there is continuous development in old age (Sherman 2010, Tornstam 2005). This theory is intended to address aging experiences of some individuals whose developmental patterns have not been addressed adequately by other theories of aging, but it is not intended to nullify other theories (Tornstam 2005). It is not intended to be a theory of "successful aging" since Tornstam considers the concept of "successful aging" problematic because "aging successfully most often is understood as continuing to be a Western-cultured, White, middle-aged, middle-class successful person, with the typical emphasis on activity, productivity, efficiency, individuality, independence, wealth, health, and sociability"(Tornstam 2005: 3). Gerotranscendence theory emphasizes change and development, and Tornstam (2005) suggests that in principle the potential for arriving at gerotranscendence is universal and culture free. Movement toward gerotranscendence is a lifelong and continuous process generated by normal living and modified by cultural patterns, but this drive is not fulfilled by everyone (Tornstam 1989, 2005).

This perspective has been identified by sociologists as critical theory (Tornstam 2005) and postmodern theory (Bengtson et al. 1996) and includes a life process that is believed to optimally end in gerotranscendence. It recalls psychologist Erik Erikson's developmental theory in which ego integrity is to be achieved in the final stage of life based on accomplishment of developmental tasks during each life stage (Tornstam 1989, 2005). However, Erikson's and Tornstam's perspectives differ because "the ego-integrity described by Erikson becomes more of a backwards integration process within the same definition of the world as before, while the process of gerotranscendence implies more of a forward or outward direction, including a qualitative redefinition of reality" (Tornstam 1997: 153).

Dimensions of gerotranscendence

Hyse and Tornstam (2009: 4) refer to gerotranscendence as "the final stage of a possible natural progression toward maturation and wisdom," and Tornstam (2011) believes that gerotranscendence results from an intrinsic drive to develop, an experience that "just happens" as a part of being human. Movement toward gerotranscendence may involve changes in the cosmic dimension, the dimension of the self, and the dimension of social and personal relationships. Based on findings in Tornstam's (2005: 187) initial qualitative study, he described developmental changes in these dimensions as follows.

The cosmic dimension

Movement toward gerotranscendence in the cosmic dimension includes developmental changes in the areas of time and childhood, connection to earlier generations, life and death, mystery in life, and rejoicing:

> *Time and childhood.* Changes in the definitions of time and the return of childhood. The transcendence of borders between past and present occurs. Childhood comes to life – sometimes interpreted in a new reconciling way.

> *Connection to earlier generations.* Attachment increases. A change in perspective from link to chain ensues. The important thing is not the individual life (link), but rather the stream of life (chain).

> *Life and death.* The fear of death disappears and a new comprehension of life and death results.

> *Mystery in life.* The mystery dimension in life is accepted.

> *Rejoicing.* From grand events to subtle experiences. The joy of experiencing the macrocosm through the microcosm materializes, not infrequently related to experiences in nature.

> (Tornstam 2005: 188)

The dimension of the self

Movement toward gerotranscendence in the dimension of the self includes changes in the areas of self-confrontation, decrease in self-centeredness, development of body transcendence, development of self-transcendence, and ego integrity:

> *Self-confrontation.* The discovery of hidden aspects of the self – both good and bad – occurs.
>
> *Decrease in self-centeredness.* Removal of the self from the center of one's universe may eventuate. However, if self-esteem from beginning is low, it may instead be a question of struggling to establish a level of confidence that feels appropriate.
>
> *Development of body-transcendence.* Taking care of the body continues, but the individual is not obsessed with it.
>
> *Self-transcendence.* A shift may occur from egoism to altruism. This may be a special matter for men.
>
> *Ego-integrity.* The individual realizes that the pieces of life's jigsaw puzzle form a wholeness. This may be a delicate state, demanding tranquility and solitude.
>
> (Tornstam 2005: 188)

The dimension of social and personal relationships

Movement toward gerotranscendence in the dimension of social and personal relationships includes changes in the areas of meaning and importance of relations, role play, emancipated innocence, modern asceticism, and everyday wisdom:

> *Changed meaning and importance of relations.* One becomes more selective and less interested in superficial relations, exhibiting an increasing need for periods of solitude.
>
> *Role play.* An understanding of the difference between self and role takes place, sometimes with an urge to abandon roles. A new, comforting understanding of the necessity of roles in life often results.
>
> *Emancipated innocence.* Innocence enhances maturity. A new capacity to transcend needless social conventions.
>
> *Modern asceticism.* An understanding of the petrifying gravity of wealth and the freedom of "asceticism" develops, i.e., having enough for a modern definition of the necessities of life, but not more.
>
> *Everyday wisdom.* The reluctance to superficially separate right from wrong, thus withholding from judgments and giving advice is discerned. Transcendence of the right-wrong duality ensues, and is accompanied by an increased broad-mindedness and tolerance
>
> (Tornstam 2005: 188–9)

Contemplative aging

Tornstam (2011) considers Edmund Sherman's conceptualization of "contemplative aging" to be consistent with gerotranscendence theory. Sherman (2010: 4) notes that dimensions in life experiences in aging that are aspects of gerotranscendence have been identified through in-depth interviews and survey research conducted primarily in Scandinavian countries and that questions can be asked about the possibility of value preferences that may differ from "the largely American conception of successful old age." However, Sherman, a retired professor of social welfare, has found that many of the elders whom he has counseled in the U.S. report transcendent experiences consistent with gerotranscendence theory and that these are "at the heart of contemplative aging" (2010: 4).

Sherman (2010: 15) suggests that a developmental shift toward contemplation involves movement from an orientation toward "being" rather than "doing" that is not regressive. Contemplation is "*doing* something," but its emergence and practice requires a change in attitude and habitual patterns of living. According to Sherman, doing and being are inseparable and innate polarities of our existence that cannot be separated existentially, and the capacity for moving toward contemplation occurs naturally as people age. However, it must be recognized and cultivated in order to be realized. This ontological shift has been described by research psychologists as a natural development of increased interiority of the personality that tends to occur around the time that people are entering their sixties. This is described as a shift from an active to passive form of mastery, and passive mastery is described by Sherman (2010: 16) as:

> ...the use of mental capacities, like memory and imagination, become more prominent in later life relative to motility and action in dealing with the environment, with one's own body, and with life's circumstances. This form of mastery is marked by increasing commitment to a central core of values and ways of behaving and relating to the outside world. At the same time, with this turn inward, many of the old attachments and animosities, likes and dislikes, alliances, grudges, and ambitions lose their hold on people. Elders feel more able to concentrate on their core values, on the cohesion and continuity of the essential elements of their personalities, and on the meaning of their lives.

While this transformative shift is less obvious in the U.S. than in cultures that recognize and support this kind of later life development, it occurs and allows emergence of inner capacities that can compensate for and transcend physical and social losses (Sherman 2010).

Empirical support for gerotranscendence theory

In 1991, Tornstam (2005: 48) conducted a qualitative phenomenological study after 50 self-selected volunteers between the ages of 52 and 97 were recruited following a lecture in which he presented tentative ideas about the theory of gerotranscendence. He asked for volunteers who "might recognize something of the ideas presented in their own personal development" and would be willing to be interviewed. Two or three volunteers thought that the developmental idea was interesting and agreed to participate in semi-structured interviews that lasted between one and three hours. In addition to qualitative research, quantitative studies that have provided empirical support for gerotranscendence include the *1990 Danish Retrospective Study* in which 912 Danish men and women between the ages of 74 and 100 responded to retrospective questions about gerotranscendence-related developments in life. The *Swedish 1995 Cross-Sectional Study* included 2,002 respondents between the ages of 20 and 85 in a mail survey. The *Swedish 2001 (65+) Study* asked questions generated from previous studies in a mail survey of 1,771 Swedish men (Tornstam 2005).

Tornstam explains that psychological strain, depression, mental insufficiency, and consumption of psychotropic medications were controlled for in the *1990 Danish Retrospective Study*, and therefore the findings could not be explained by these factors. However, he suggests that consumption of psychotropic medications might interfere with achievement of gerotranscendence (Tornstam 2005).

Results from the 1995 and 2001 studies indicate that cosmic transcendence and coherence are processes that develop continuously beginning during the first half of adult life and achieve maximum development in later life. Need for solitude appears to develop most rapidly during the first half of adult life and increase to a maximum in late life. The research indicated that participants at the upper end of the age scale who experienced more cosmic transcendence and coherence experienced more satisfaction with life. The combination of cosmic transcendence and enhanced life satisfaction appeared to be a combination experienced especially in old age. Although these are important findings, Tornstam believes that it is important to consider limitations related to the cross-sectional research approach and cultural and temporal limitations of these studies in Sweden (Tornstam 2005: 190).

According to Tornstam, these findings indicate that life circumstances, or social-matrix factors, are important influences in development of cosmic transcendence in young and middle-aged people. Life crises positively influenced development of cosmic transcendence in both women and men who participated in the studies, and students and people with self-governed professions scored higher in this dimension. However, age had greater explanatory power for men since age had twice as much explanatory power as crises. Tornstam found that crises appeared to have less impact on development of cosmic transcendence in old age. Women scored higher than men in cosmic transcendence from ages 20 to 64, but men's and women's scores were similar at age 75 and older (Tornstam 2005).

Social matrix and incident impact predictors, including lack of crises, high activity, being married, and former qualified profession, appeared to be related to greater coherence. In old age, pure positive age development and social-matrix and incident impact factors appeared to equally determine experiences of coherence.

This could affect a person's preexisting degree of coherence either positively or negatively. The causes of need for solitude as an attribute of gerotranscendence appeared to be age-related developmental change and reactions to incident-impact factors like crises and diseases (Tornstam 2005).

Jannie Pevik Fasth (2007, 2011) and Barbro Wadensten (2005, 2007, 2010; Wadensten and Hagglund 2006; Wadensten and Carlsson 2007a; Wadensten and Carlsson 2007b) have researched use of especially designed social work and nursing approaches in Sweden that have been developed to support development of gerotranscendence in older adults. Social worker Pevik Fasth conducted a study in Hudiksvall, Sweden, to investigate whether basic knowledge of gerotranscendence theory among healthcare workers visiting elders in their homes could improve the quality of the preventive healthcare interviews that they conducted. This was a comparative study in which three healthcare workers were given information about gerotranscendence and conducted qualitative interviews that included questions based on gerotranscendence theory. The second group of healthcare workers was limited to using an inquiry form developed by the Swedish Health and Human Services Department (*Socialstyrelsen*) and not given information about gerotranscendence. Pevik Fasth and Brandt (2007: 1) concluded that:

> the interviews which included the theory of Gerotranscendence in a wider sense created an atmosphere consisting of emotional safeness, a deeper personal connection and mutual understanding. The elders also seemed to react positively to the opportunity to talk about their psychosocial development and to get a chance to talk about the deeper philosophical questions of life.

Pevik Fasth (2011) also participated in a research study in which life development groups for older people between the ages of 80 and 90 met every second week for more than six months and were interviewed before and after the study period. The content included information about the domains of gerotranscendence theory, and all participants experienced development toward gerotranscendence in at least some domains. At the end of the study, the older adults could recognize more aspects of gerotranscendence as a result of exploring the concept of gerotranscendence, including looking more deeply into gerotranscendent change. Pevik Fasth notes that it is difficult to find these aspects of oneself because of society's negative attitudes about aging and older adults and because people are not talking about these changes. Because achievement of gerotranscendence involves taking time to withdraw from interaction with others, people may not understand and this can be a difficult process if there is lack of support (Pevik Fasth 2011).

Pevik Fasth (2011) also facilitates development of gerotranscendence in older adults as a social worker in her municipality's Hudiksvall Whole Life program. She integrates gerotranscendence theory into her work with the life development group for older adults age 75 and over who were participants in the research study and with whom she has continued to work. Group members have continued to discuss their life stories and explore their inner selves. Pevik Fasth is also recruiting volunteers in Hudiksvall to learn about the dimensions of gerotranscendence, experience their own journey into gerotranscendence, and then learn to facilitate gerotranscendence groups in nursing homes and locations in the community where older people gather. She has also developed a monthly talk show in Hudiksvall from the gerotranscendence perspective and a collaborative effort of four agencies to change attitudes about aging through use of this perspective. This project includes speaking with politicians about the importance of gerotranscendence.

Barbro Wadensten has written about application of this theoretical perspective in nursing research and practice to support development of gerotranscendence in older adults. Wadensten (2007: 292) considers gerotranscendence theory to be different from other theories of aging because "it defines a reality somewhat different from the middle-age reality and lifestyle. Other theories of ageing are often based on the assumption that 'successful ageing' implies retaining the activities and ideals of middle age." According to Wadensten and Carlsson (2007a), nursing staff has been trained to think that all older people should become active regardless of whether this is the preference of the older person. With the goal of supporting development of nursing practice that facilitates growth and sustainment of gerotranscendence in older people, Wadensten and Carlsson (2007a, 2007b) developed guidelines to be used as a supplement to enrich nursing care of older people. These can also be useful to older adults themselves, family members, friends, and service providers in other fields to support development of gerotranscendence in older adults. The guidelines include specific approaches for nurses to use:

(1) focus on the individual with an understanding that behaviors resembling gerotranscendence are normal in aging; (2) reduce preoccupation with the body by initiating conversation about topics other than health or physical limitations; (3) allow alternative definitions of time, inquiring about the person's past adventures and respecting the reality that older people perceive time differently; (4) allow thoughts and conversations about death and address the subject of death when a person who the older adult knows has died; (5) choose topics of conversation that facilitate and further older people's personal growth, including discussion of feelings, dreams, their childhood, and life development; (6) focus on acceptance, creation, and introduction of activities supporting gerotranscendence; and (7) address organization by encouraging and facilitating the older person's opportunities for peace and quiet.

(Wadensten and Carlsson 2007a: 297)

Implementing these guidelines, Wadensten and Carlsson (2007b) conducted research in which the theory of gerotranscendence and the guidelines were taught to a convenience sample of nursing staff in a nursing home. "Early adopters" of the perspective were staff for whom essential ideas in the theory were familiar since they believed that they were engaged in a personal developmental process consistent with the theory. Other participants had more difficulty changing their interpretations, values, and treatment of older people. Results were analyzed from the perspective of Rogers's innovation attributes that are considered most important in adoption of an innovation: "1. Observability (visibility); 2. Relative advantage associated with using it; 3. Lack of complexity (understandability); 4. Compatibility with extant values; 5. Trialability (potential to be acquired 'piece by piece') (Wadensten and Carlsson 2007b: 303).

Findings indicated that Rogers's innovation theory was useful but lacked another important attribute, the "aha-experience" of some of the nurses. Other findings included changes in many nurses' descriptions of residents' behavior that was previously interpreted as "pathological" to descriptions of behavior as "normal" following the intervention, increased recognition of signs and acceptance of residents by staff after the intervention, and increased use of gerotranscendence guidelines by staff who recognized signs of gerotranscendence before intervention and considered these signs to be "normal." Findings from participant observation and qualitative interviews with six residents indicated that staff changed the topics of conversations with the residents which led to more reflective discussions between staff and residents, and staff encouraged and helped residents to have quiet and peaceful time. However, it cannot be assumed that residents' increased reflectiveness was dependent only on the gerotranscendence intervention (Wadensten 2010).

In Wadensten's (2005) qualitative study in a day center, the intervention consisted of group sessions with female participants who discussed their aging and viewed a video about the theory of gerotranscendence and discussed its relationship to their experiences of growing old. The participants considered introduction to gerotranscendence theory to be beneficial because of its positive view of aging. Wadensten and Hagglund (2006) describe a more recent study in a day center in which eight men and women between the ages of 74 and 85 were divided into two groups to participate in reminiscence groups with the goals of development, reorganization, and change in their identity. During the eight weeks of group participation intended to encourage and support the process toward gerotranscendence, the nurse leader guided discussion that addressed intended themes and helped participants to reflect. Between five and six weeks after the conclusion, another nurse interviewed the participants about their experiences. Participants had experienced their group very differently, with female participants experiencing it more reflectively, and Wadensten and Hagglund (2006) note that culture can facilitate or impede the process of gerotranscendence.

Tornstam (2011) believes that more work needs to be done to learn about cultural contrasts in gerotranscendence experiences. Cultural diversity is reflected in a study about gerotranscendence and life satisfaction among religious and secular Iranians and Turks (Ahmadi Lewin and Thomas 2000); research in Japan about life narratives of people 85 and older (Nakagawa et al. 2011) and use of a gerotranscendence questionnaire (Masui et al. 2010); cosmic transcendence, loneliness, and exchange of emotional support with adult children in a study of older adults in the Netherlands (Sadler et al. 2006); and studies in the U.S. about people 85 and older in the San Francisco Bay area (Shaskan 2009) and older adults in Florida belonging to diverse racial and ethnic groups (Nobles 2010).

Fereshteh Ahmadi Lewin's (2000) cross-cultural analysis of Iranian older adults living in Sweden and Turks residing in Turkey is a culturally comparative study to determine whether there is any relationship between gerotranscendence and life satisfaction. This analysis is based on an international research study by Lars Tornstam, Fereshteh Ahmadi Lewin, and L. Eugene Thomas to analyze late life development of religious and secular individuals from the perspectives of gerotranscendence and spiritual development. The study devoted particular attention to intermingled factors of belief-induced developmental patterns and developmental patterns connected with universal archetypal processes of aging. The goal was "to determine the applicability of the theory [Theory of Gerotranscendence] in as many different cultural settings as possible, and with groups known to hold allegiance to cultural goals differing from that of main-stream society" (Thomas 1997: 1, in Ahmadi Lewin 2000: 18). An additional objective was to study whether people who demonstrated evidence of gerotran-scendence also showed evidence of life satisfaction. Life stories and stories of self-development of secular and religious older adults in Turkey who were between the ages of 66 and 83 were deconstructed and compared with life stories and self-development of Iranian immigrants in Sweden. The Iranian respondents immigrated to Sweden after the Islamic Revolution and were between the ages of 43 and 75 at the time of their interviews. All of the religious older people in Ahmadi Lewin's analysis were Sufi Muslims. Sufis were included as the main religious group "since their goal is to develop their perception of self as well as their social and individual relationships into a 'way of thinking' that seems to have connections to both the Theory of Gerotranscendence and to L.E. Thomas' study about elderly people's spiritual maturity" (Ahmadi Lewin 2000: 18).

Interview transcripts were coded in eight dimensions of gerotranscendence: (1) view of time and space; (2) view of life and death; (3) self-understanding; (4) decrease in self-centeredness; (5) transcendent wisdom; (6) meaning and importance of relations; (7) mystery dimension of life; and (8) attitude toward material assets (Ahmadi Lewin 2000: 23–4). Analysis of interview content used an hermeneutical approach in which it was assumed that a subtext must be under-stood in light of the entire text and the entire text understood in terms of the components in order to truly understand the text. The researchers read the inter-view protocols independently and engaged with their own assumptions resulting from their individual histories of prior research and/or personal and cultural knowledge. They discussed their analyses and returned to the original protocols to ensure that identified meaning units were firmly grounded in the data (Ahmadi Lewin 2000: 25–7).

Findings from the Turkish interviews indicated that some respondents demon-strated clear evidence of gerotranscendence while others, including people who were considered very religious, were found to be almost completely lacking in gerotranscendence. Evidence of life satisfaction was demonstrated by all people in the sample who demonstrated gerotranscendence: a "more accurate description would be to say they radiated a remarkable sense of contentment in their lives, and a keen appreciation of life" (Ahmadi Lewin 2000: 27). However, there were respondents, especially in the secular sample, who showed no evidence of gerotranscendence, "yet a great zest for life, satisfaction with their past accomplishments, and acceptance of their past without regret" (Ahmadi Lewin 2000: 28).

Responses in the Iranian interviews showed evidence of gerotranscendence among both religious and secular persons, and these individuals also demonstrated evidence of life satisfaction. The relationship was more apparent in the sample of religious people. Results from the Iranian respondents differed from Turkish responses because some Turkish respondents demonstrated evidence of life satisfaction without gerotranscendence (Ahmadi Lewin 2000: 28, 30, 37).

Ahmadi Lewin (2000: 38-9) concludes that analysis of data from the interviews with Iranian and Turkish respondents supports the hypothesis of a positive relationship between gerotranscendence and life satisfaction but that it should not be assumed that a gerotranscendent world view is necessary for achieving life satisfaction. There were Turkish respondents who showed evidence of life satisfaction without evidence of gerotranscendence in spite of major challenges including loss of spouse, financial limitations, and health problems. Ahmadi Lewin (2000: 39) concludes by asserting that "there is neither a 'universal' mystical experience nor a 'universal' gerotranscendent experience, but that these are instead dependent on the individual's cultural and religious tradition as well as social circumstances."

Research example: case study of a gerotranscendent older adult

Karin Hyse and Lars Tornstam (2009) describe a single subject research study in Sweden that focused on Mary, a woman who identified aspects of herself in the theory of gerotranscendence after learning about the theory from a brief presentation by Tornstam on a Swedish television program. She e-mailed her observations to Tornstam, and Hyse followed up with in-depth interviews when Mary was 75 years old. Although Hyse and Tornstam (2009: 5) understand that reported identification with a theory can be "reconstructions of reality or rationalizations that allow older people to align their lived lives with a pleasant, hopeful theory," they believe that Mary's experiences are consistent with the theory because she shared relevant material that she had written about her experiences prior to learning about gerotranscendence theory.

During the first interview session, Mary freely provided a narrative description about her entire life, and a biographical thematic interview followed. A question guide that focused on the theory of gerotranscendence was used in the second interview, and there was informal discussion after each of the formal interviews ended. Hyse also read excerpts from diaries and booklets that Mary had written for her children, relatives, and friends. At the time of the interviews, Mary was very happy about her situation. She lived alone in a medium-sized town in northern Sweden, was in close contact with her children and grandchildren, had retired at age 60 after employment in several professions, experienced good health except for a disease causing chronic pain, and did not demonstrate signs of psychological disturbance or dementia (Hyse and Tornstam 2009).

In their description and interpretation of Mary's narrative as it relates to gerotranscendence, Hyse and Tornstam used two interpretive tools, the first of which is the "mountain climber metaphor." This metaphorical thinking about gerotranscendence theory stimulated their reasoning during analysis of the verbal and written information provided by Mary. The mountain climber metaphor provides a view of "life as a mountain that we climb over the course of our life" (Hyse and Tornstam 2009: 7).

The second interpretive tool was a "typology of ways of life" based on Oberg's (1997) typology that Hyse and Tornstam believed might be useful for developing understanding of how Mary had reached gerotranscendence. Oberg has defined a "way of life" as: "[…] the strategy an individual uses to take advantage of the resources created by social background, education, tradition and the market" (Oberg 1997: 38, translation by Hyse and Tornstam, in Hyse and Tornstam 2009: 7). Hyse and Tornstam (2009: 8) explain:

> Based on the oral life narratives provided by a number of elderly people, Oberg was able to identify six types of life narratives – ways of life – that also show how events from the entire life course are mirrored in old age:
>
> *The Bitter Life:* A life full of tragedies and losses. A difficult childhood without basic security and lacking in any real contact with one's parents. Poor adult relationships with one's partner and other people. Health problems leading to difficulties in functioning in everyday life. Life did not turn out at all as one had thought. In old age, one has become depressed and isolated, lacking any positive belief in the future.
>
> *Life as a Trapping Pit:* A life that begins with a troubled childhood. Later in life, one has either been married, but often without children, or had a very dysfunctional marriage. During the life course, particularly the latter part of life, one has experienced various losses and sees oneself as a loser. One has experienced one pitfall after another, and life did not turn out as one had imagined it would. One has no positive belief in the future.
>
> *Life as a Hurdle Race:* Life begins with losses and problems in childhood. Other problems continue, e.g., marriage difficulties, too many children, illnesses, alcohol problems, poor relationships with other people. But one sees oneself as a fighter who can overcome any difficulty and come out a winner, which paves the way for a brighter old age. Relationships with children and friends are good, and one has a positive attitude toward life as an older person.

The Devoted Silenced Life: Life is dominated by taking care of others. One has remained unmarried and without children, and has instead devoted oneself to taking care of others, e.g., one's own parents. One is nevertheless satisfied with one's life in general and experiences a pleasant old age.

Life as a Career: This way of life is predominantly experienced by men, often unmarried, who have been totally engrossed in their work or who have a family that supported their career. They define themselves through their work. They are satisfied with their life, experience a pleasant old age, and even have a positive attitude about the future.

The Sweet Life: Life begins with an idyllic childhood and continues with good health, a happy marriage and wonderful children. One is likely to have an academic degree. One has certainly had difficult times, but nothing has occurred that could not be resolved. One experiences a pleasant old age and has a positive attitude about the future.

Mary's experiences with cosmic dimensions of gerotranscendence

In their consideration of the developmental change of "Time and childhood – time and space melt together and become one" as this relates to Mary's experiences, Hyse and Tornstam (2009: 10–11) explain that Mary recognizes changes in her definition of time and space. Mary had begun to experience increasing difficulty in remembering when she had most recently seen a given person and how long ago events occurred, but she attributed this to lack of interest in these matters rather than forgetfulness. She described changes:

> Time stops. The past, present and future become one. It's not memories, do you understand? It's something strange, time and space don't exist, and everything exists now.

Mary had begun to think about and reevaluate her childhood, a development consistent with gerotranscendence:

> Memories have appeared, I don't know if they can be products of my imagination too, but I know the kind of memories you always have with you. But then I've questioned what memory is, how much do we recreate our memories? But I've thought a lot, and that's what's caused me to reevaluate my childhood.

When she began to write about her childhood five or six years before the interviews, she became aware of memories that were previously unknown to her:

> Memories appeared that I didn't think existed. And yes, it was a grieving process really. Even with the old memories in some way and I thought: how could my mother have been so goddamn nasty?

Mary's childhood was sorrowful and isolated, but she did not want her mother to read what she had written. When her mother did read what Mary had written and told her how unhappy she had been since reading this, Mary reacted:

> Then I thought, good gracious! It made me go back and think of it in a different way and I asked myself: what part do I have in all of this?

Mary decided to assume more responsibility in her relationship with her mother, their relationship improved, and Mary reported the following conversation:

> Mama, it says so in the booklet, but the fact is that I've recently started reevaluating things and then I've thought that maybe it was supposed to be like this. Actually, compared to many others I've met, I'm very happy in my old age. I feel my life is rich and meaningful.[...]

Mary continued to be angry at her mother, but developed understanding that her mother may have done the best that she could. She became grateful for her difficult childhood because her experiences had given her the capacity for empathy for people experiencing sorrow and unhappiness (Hyse and Tornstam 2009: 11).

Mary appeared to be developing gerotranscendence in other cosmic dimensions: related to experiencing connection to earlier generations, she had begun to research her genealogy several years before. Related to the dimension of disappearance of fear of death and new comprehension of life and death, she said: "In one way, I think life is terribly exciting and great fun, but in another way I could give it up. That's pretty paradoxical." Hyse and Tornstam interpret Mary's uniting of these two ideas as evidence of progress in gerotranscendental development (Hyse and Tornstam 2009: 12–13).

Mary described herself as previously a very analytical person who wanted everything to exist in an intellectual, comprehensible, and rational pattern. However, in recent years her perspective had changed in the direction of the cosmic development in accepting the mysterious aspects of life. She told Hyse (2005: 13):

> I think like this: why waste your time trying to find explanations when you can simply live?! I can choose to sit around and think about how matters stand with my strange experiences. It might depend on this or that, but is it possible to find an explanation? I've come to one conclusion: the explanation I arrive at will certainly be wrong anyway. I say, life is marvelous, that explanation is enough for me these days. I can't solve the riddle. I just see life's wonderful beauty.

However, she valued her experiences questioning and searching for truth when she was younger:

I think maybe certain experiences are necessary, also pondering, thinking, analyzing, and searching, but then there comes a time when you have to let go of the search, because then you've experienced that you can't find the truth anyway. But everything I've read and thought is gathered together in one big experience.

Mary also experiences development towards gerotranscendence that is consistent with the theory's description of "how causes for *rejoicing* change from grand events to subtle experiences, and how the joy of experiencing the micro cosmos in the macro cosmos materializes, often related to experiences in nature." Hyse and Tornstam (2009: 13–14) explain:

A great change has occurred in what Mary appreciates in life and in what makes her happy, for instance she traveled a great deal. At present, Mary has no need to visit the neighboring town, but can experience happiness in relation to small events. These could be everyday encounters in town with people she knows or does not know. Music and nature are two of her greatest joys. Mary spends at least two hours a day listening to music, and she has an allotment she loves to be in:
Birds, plants, trees, they don't just please me – they make me happy. Music makes me happy.

Mary also tells about a woman friend who travels all over the world, but who still says she does not feel life has anything exciting to offer. Mary's reaction is as follows:

Are you crazy? I think going to the grocery store is exciting.

Just as described in the theory of gerotranscendence, Mary's causes for joy in life have changed, from rather extravagant traveling to subtle everyday events.

Mary's experiences with the dimension of the self

Self-confrontation, reduced self-centeredness, self-transcendence, and ego-integrity are all dimensions of the self in which Mary is moving toward gerotranscendence (Hyse and Tornstam 2009: 14–16). She had become more aware in recent years of both negative and positive aspects of herself and had developed greater self-confidence and acceptance of herself:

I've had poor self-confidence, but now when I've grown older, it's like a fiasco doesn't bother me as much anymore. Sometimes I think I can't do this. But then I get started and realize that I actually can accomplish things. […] Unthinkable ten years ago!

The following statement in which she compared her sense of self-importance to her earlier life reflects reduced self-centeredness that is consistent with gerotranscendent development:

> Less important because I'm just a little speck in the universe. [...] A little grain, so in that sense I'm not important in the slightest. But at the same time I notice that I do important things. So it's both really.

Mary's process of development of self-transcendence in the sense of a change from egoism to altruism was described by Hyse and Tornstam (2009: 15): "she has become in a sense more egocentric and less egoistic. By more egocentric she means that when she sees friends and family, she talks a good deal about her life and what is happening around her. Mary believes this is because she has no partner to share daily experiences with. But during recent years, she feels she primarily does things to please others.

> That's why what gives me most joy is to feel that what I do will be of benefit to others and to see other people's happiness. [...] And then sometimes I think, what is egoism really, isn't it egoistic to rejoice in other people's joy? Yes, but I don't care, I don't care if egoism is behind it or not because here on earth we don't know if it's egoism being non-egoistic or maybe just as egoistic.

Development of ego integrity is reflected in her gratitude for what she has been given in life: "now, when she looks at her life as a whole, it feels like the puzzle pieces have come together and she experiences coherence."

The sole dimension in which Mary does not appear to have achieved gerotranscendence is body transcendence. She has continued her lifelong pattern of neglecting her body:

> Yes, there I fall short. I should take better care, I know. I should be wiser, get more exercise and eat healthier food and so on. [...] I know that I'd be able to do more if my body was in better shape, but I still neglect it, which isn't good.

She is critical about her appearance but said that she no longer cares as much about her looks (Hyse and Tornstam 2009: 15).

Mary's experiences with the dimension of social and personal relationships

Mary's experiences were consistent with movement toward gerotranscendence in all areas in this dimension (Hyse and Tornstam 2009: 16–18). Solitude and silence became more important, transcendence of needless social conventions and increased tendency toward impulsiveness, greater understanding of self and role and urge to abandon roles, and modern asceticism: "understanding of the petrifying gravity of excessive wealth" as well as movement toward a new perspective of "having enough for a modern definition of the necessities of life, but no more" had occurred. Related to modern asceticism:

> Mary says that her need to buy clothes and other objects has diminished a great deal during recent years. Earlier, she could buy expensive clothes and other items, but now she would rather give away things she feels she no longer needs. Although her personal economy is not exceptionally good, she is not worried because she knows she will always have enough money for her food and rent. She thinks that is enough now and she explains it by saying:
>
> My financial situation is worse than before, it's pretty bad actually. I've got some savings and a pension, but it gets worse and worse with every year that passes, because my [sic] I'm using up my savings. But I think: I've got my pension, I've got enough to buy food and I will be able to live here in the future.

Mary has experienced decreased interest in superficial relationships, and her relationships with her closest friends have deepened. Her need for contacts with other people is balanced with her need for solitude:

> Before I thought I needed solitude so I could digest things. Think about why life turned out like it did and things like that and how I wanted life to be now. But now, solitude is just solitude and silence, it's not filled up with so many thoughts or pondering about what it was like when I was a child or what I'll do tomorrow. Not for reflecting on life so much any more, but just for enjoying and being in silence. I mean, you always have thoughts, but there's a difference.

Mary no longer wants to play roles; she describes herself as trying to be who she is, and she also values her gerotranscedent behavior of mature emancipated innocence in which spontaneity has been added to her mature personality.

Mary's development of everyday wisdom is also consistent with gerotranscendence and is indicated by the fact that she has learned that bad decisions may lead to something good. The theory states that with gerotranscendence "the certainty of youth about what is right or wrong diminishes and...insights into the fluidness of boundaries develops." According to Mary,

> When you look back at your life, you find that often, often, it's the incorrect choices that have led to a happier and more meaningful life.

Hyse and Tornstam add that "Mary asks herself why, at this point, she would know the truth, when she has changed her opinions on different matters several times during her life and will probably change them again very soon" (Hyse and Tornstam 2009: 18).

Hyse and Tornstam's analysis of Mary's narrative

Hyse and Tornstam (2009) analyzed Mary's narrative from the perspectives of Oberg's life course typification and the mountain climber metaphor with particular emphasis on the themes of crises and turning points, social relations, reevaluations, and old age. Mary's major life crises appeared to have been the crisis throughout her entire childhood when her mother sent her away from home at times, the crisis when a man left Mary, a crisis when she ended a relationship with a man who she could not be involved with even though she loved him deeply and, although Mary did not consider this to be major, her contraction of a disease causing severe pain. Hyse and Tornstam (2009: 20) note that Arvidsson has proposed that the important events in a narrative are the turning points, and they regard each of these events to be turning points despite the fact that Mary's collective childhood experiences were not a single delimited crisis event. Mary's history of overcoming crises, receiving positive benefits from these experiences, and retaking control is identified by Hyse and Tornstam (2009) as consistent with Oberg's "life as a hurdle race" life course type.

In Mary's narrative, thematic content pertaining to social relations centers on love for the men she has met, friends, children, and grandchildren, as well as relationships with developmentally disabled people who she has met through her volunteer work. Hyse and Tornstam (2009: 21) suggest that Mary's strong connections to people with developmental disabilities may be related to her progress in her gerotranscendent development. Her experiences with these individuals and their views of the world may have opened her mind to different outlooks and created a foundation for her own reevaluation of life.

Mary's narrative reflects openness to reinterpretations and reevaluations in life that are consistent with gerotranscendental development (Hyse and Tornstam 2009: 21–2):

> Mary's own spontaneous life narrative starts in her childhood. She describes how she grew up in an environment with trees, a hammock and a lovely view of a lake. The beginning of the story seemed to promise a description of a most ideal childhood, but that did not turn out to be the case. Mary instead describes how mean her mother was, how her father hit her and how she was sent away from her home for a period when she was a toddler because her mother felt she did not have time for two children. Mary reports that she has always hated her mother and that she does so to this day. But she also says that her views on her childhood and her relationship with her mother have changed during recent years. Mary has realized that it may be because of her horrible childhood that she has been given the gift of feeling strong empathy with other people. If she were given the chance today to choose another childhood, she would not change things, which she told her mother:
>
> > Mama, my childhood may be the best thing that could've happened to me, because thanks to it I'm able to understand other people's

deep sorrow and unhappiness. [...] If I could choose now and got to have a happy and harmonious childhood, I'd still choose the same one.

Earlier in life, Mary wished she had had a different and happier childhood, but this has changed, and her reinterpretation and reevaluation also include an element of reconciliation with her horrible childhood mother, though Mary reports still hating her mother.

This interesting reevaluation of childhood may be more understandable if we consider the mountain climber metaphor. Only when Mary has climbed high up on the mountain and can look back on her terrible childhood is she able to see that it has entailed something good. She sees how her childhood has helped her to find paths that let her help other people, who perhaps have been of help to her during difficult times.

According to Hyse and Tornstam (2009: 22), openness to reinterpretations and reevaluations is important in gerotranscendental development. They write that in her narrative "Mary shows that she has dared to let go of previous valuations and has been open to seeing earlier events and valuations in a new light and from the perspective of the entire lived life – as seen from the top of life's mountain."

Summary

Gerotranscendence theory was developed by Swedish sociologist Lars Tornstam as a meta-theoretical reformulation of disengagement theory. Tornstam asserts that disengagement is a positive movement toward gerotranscendence that can be followed by increased life satisfaction. Gerotranscendence theory asserts that the character, values, and meaning of old age are different from the attributes of the middle age years and there is continuous development in old age. Movement toward gerotranscendence may involve changes in the cosmic dimension, the dimension of the self, and the dimension of social and personal relationships. Tornstam considers U.S. social worker Edmund Sherman's theory of contemplative aging to be consistent with gerotranscendence theory.

According to Tornstam, this theory represents a positive shift in meta-perspective to a more cosmic and transcendent view compared to a materialistic and rational view. In the case example based on Thornstam and Hyse's research in Sweden, Hyse's description of "Mary" provides examples of achievement of gerotranscendence in each of these dimensions. There have been applications of gerotranscendence theory in applied practice fields and research. In Sweden, Jannie Pevik Fasth and Barbro Wadensten have researched and applied gerotranscendence theory in therapeutic approaches to gerontological service provision in their respective fields of social work and nursing.

The question of whether there is a relationship between gerotranscendence and life satisfaction has been studied in cross-cultural research by Tornstam, Ahmadi Lewin, and Thomas. Findings indicated that life satisfaction can exist without achievement of gerotranscendence and that life satisfaction can be achieved when gerotranscendence exists. Tornstam believes that additional research about gerotranscendence theory in different cultural contexts is needed. He believes that the transformative shift is less obvious in the U.S. than in cultures that recognize and support this kind of later life development, but it occurs and allows emergence of inner capacities that can compensate for and transcend physical and social losses. Edmund Sherman has written about gerotranscendence and has known older adults in the U.S. who are gerotranscendent.

8 Theory, diversity, and policy

Key concepts

1. Richard Settersten and Molly Trauten assert that in the twenty-first century all of human experience appears to be in flux, and they identify emerging hallmarks of aging and "shifting sands and mines" that create opportunities and risks for older adults and opportunities for theoretical advances and empirical investigation.

2. Settersten and Trauten consider altered terms of life, illness, and death; individualization of old age; new freedoms and risks in old age; and old age as a highly contingent period to be new and emerging hallmarks of old age.

3. "Shifting sands" in the lives of older adults include revolutions in cohort composition and experiences and consideration of past, present, and future cohorts.

4. Fernando Torres-Gil's theoretical framework explains the politics of aging in ethnically and racially diverse societies and the influence of the intersection of race, ethnicity, politics, and old age on public policy.

5. Torres-Gil proposes that these intersections form a nexus of aging and diversity and are important to consider because demographic trends of societal aging, increasing diversity, immigration and migration, and potential political activism by older people will contribute to an emerging politics of aging consistent with his theoretical perspective.

6. Torres-Gil asserts that in his nexus model the element of diversity, otherwise known as an age-race stratified society, must be present.

7. A systematic analysis of applicability of this theory to other nations requires determination of whether the nation has aspects of racial, cultural, ethnic, and immigration diversity and whether immigration exists that could intersect with aging; evidence that organizing by older people is occurring; and whether the political systems and public policies are susceptible to a politics of aging.

8. Swedish gerontologist Mats Thorslund and U.S. gerontologist Merril Silverstein have developed a theoretical framework for analysis and prediction of global trends in public policies addressing aging under contemporary pressures of globalization.

9. They observe that most Western societies have retrenched social welfare programs in efforts to shift responsibility for assistance for older people from governments to individuals and families.
10. Thorslund and Silverstein conclude that demography is not destiny for the welfare state but may require a detour compatible with a nation's character.
11. Many organizations, including the United Nations and the World Health Organization, are addressing challenges experienced by older adults and their families globally and responding to concerns reflected in predictions of theorists and researchers about challenges to existing social welfare policies.

Introduction

Chapter 8 introduces three theoretical perspectives that address policy development in diverse societies: Richard Settersten and Molly Trauten's explanation of emerging hallmarks of aging and their implications for advances in theory and research, Fernando Torres-Gil's theoretical framework for analysis of politics of aging in societies with cultural diversity, and Thorslund and Silverstein's analysis of theories, policies, and realities of assistance for older adults in the welfare state. Torres-Gil's perspective includes application of his framework to the United States and South Korea and discussion of applicability to other nations. Description of Thorslund and Silverstein's theoretical perspectives includes comparative analysis of Sweden as a social democratic welfare state and the United States as a liberal welfare state. This chapter concludes with the subject of global advocacy for policies for the well-being of older people and describes the United Nations *Political Declaration and Madrid International Plan of Action on Aging* and related activities and the World Health Organization Global Age-friendly Cities Initiative.

Theoretical perspectives on aging policy and diversity

Emerging hallmarks of aging creating opportunities and risks for older adults

Richard Settersten and Molly Trauten (2009: 455) assert that in the twenty-first century all of human experience appears to be in flux, and they identify emerging hallmarks of aging and "shifting sands and mines" that create opportunities and risks for older adults and are ripe for theoretical advances and empirical investigation. They suggest that there are important opportunities to rethink theories of aging: "what can be kept, what must be recast, what must be discarded, and what might be created anew to do better by the complexities of aging and old people in a complicated world" (Settersten and Trauten 2009: 456). Settersten and Trauten (2009: 456–8) have identified new and emerging hallmarks of old age:

1. altered terms of life, illness, and death;
2. the individualization of old age;

3. new freedoms and risks in old age;
4. the big "ifs": old age as a highly contingent period.

Implications of emerging hallmarks for developing theory and research

Addressing the hallmarks of altered terms of life, illness, and death, Settersten and Trauten (2009: 456) point out that these changes have transformed human experiences and created aging societies over the past century with the result of creating a "longer, healthier landscape" for old age. Therefore, individuals can experience later adulthood in new ways. The decades of old age have early and late phases that can be very different, and a long and healthy life has become increasingly likely. There is a trend toward compression of morbidity in which chronic illness is increasingly confined to old age and often followed quickly by death. However, it is apparent that these trends do not occur universally throughout the world.

Settersten and Trauten (2009) propose that theories of aging could be revolutionized by the demographic imperative of life in a society where there are many old people, and particularly many older women, and attention should be given to the ways that the demographic parameters producing aging societies reverberate in all life periods, as well as in old age. Consistent with Riley and Riley's (1986) concept of structural lag, Settersten and Trauten (2009: 456) indicate the importance of exploring the ways that social institutions and policies guiding and governing every sphere of life may "lag behind the times and need to be rearchitected" to reflect demographic changes.

Addressing the hallmark of individualization of old age, Settersten and Trauten (2009) note the reality that there have been changes since the mid-twentieth century in traditional timetables related to timing and sequence of role transitions in the areas of education, work, retirement, and family. They (2009: 457) suggest that there has been "proliferation of a wide range of timetables, and even the elimination of timetables altogether." They also point out that while there is identification of individual behavior and ambitions in old age that defy age-based expectations, there is lack of clarity about exactly what constitutes age-based expectations. Settersten and Trauten (2009: 457) suggest that:

> It seems easier to recognize the things that shatter our assumptions than to recognize the things that fit and be fully aware of the assumptions we take for granted – whether in our everyday lives or in theories and research on aging. So what is it that we assume individuals are to be doing or striving for in old age? How are these decades to be filled? Is it that there are no scripts for old age, few scripts, or new scripts that are in the process of being developed?
>
> Age...has become a poor predictor of self-concepts, of achievements or failures, of the anticipations of things yet to come, and of capacities to cope with change. The task of theorizing about old age becomes more difficult when these decades are understood to be highly variable and unstable leaving little regularity to describe or explain.

Settersten and Trauten raise additional issues that have implications for advances in theory and research. They assert that existing theories of aging and the life course offer little insight into what people of a particular age or life period share, have in common as a group or as individuals, across the decades of old age. They also suggest that existing theories have little to say about what marks movement from one life period to the next. Settersten and Trauten (2009: 457) suggest that:

> Perhaps nowhere is the degree of variability among people in an age-group greater than it is among old people, as individuals' life experiences over at least six decades of adulthood culminate in what seem like personalized constellations of experiences that are as unique as one's fingerprints. The highly individualized routes taken through old age presumably only exacerbate the variability we would already expect to find among old people. Yet some things about late life, such as normative declines in physical and cognitive health, may be postponed but not escaped. In this sense, becoming and being old can also come with a set of common experiences that are often deemphasized...

The hallmark identified as new freedoms and risks in old age relates to the flexibility to live life in ways congruent with personal interests and wishes, but new risks accompany new freedoms. Settersten and Trauten (2009: 457–8) highlight diversity of experiences when they suggest that for old people the future seems "fragile, unpredictable, dwindling, and compressed," as well as open:

> Choices now seem greater, but these choices may also seem heavier and come with unknown consequences. Any fallouts must also be negotiated and absorbed by individuals and their families rather than by governments, markets, or other entities (at least in the context of American policy). The trend toward individualization means that old people are increasingly left to their own devices to determine the directions that the ends of their lives will take. Old people are largely on their own with only the safety nets they can create with the resources they have, whether through personal and family resources or through social skills and psychological capacities.

Settersten and Trauten (2009: 458) suggest that pursuit of new pathways by older people that are not widely shared with others or reinforced by institutions or policies may lead to loss of sources of formal and informal support. These theorists (2009: 458) suggest that it is important to "redefine and broaden thinking about the groups of people who are at risk as they move through life – and, in the case of old age, arrive with long histories of risk that greatly influence the freedoms or constraints that individuals feel during life's final decades." Loss of support can have especially negative effects on individuals and groups already at risk since they may have less time to recover and fewer personal and social resources, and policies based on outdated models of life may harm them. The lack of clear scripts for life has the potential to affect the mental health of individuals because of the lack of a shared framework to assess themselves and others. Settersten and Trauten (2009: 458) ask:

> How can people make plans, set goals, and take action, knowing all the while that their lives will be continually altered in ways that cannot be predicted and can be only partially controlled? What are the implications for how societies might function when age-based norms vanish? These are central challenges for theorizing aging and the life course in postindustrial societies.

For theorists of aging, Settersten and Trauten (2009: 458) indicate that:

> No matter how such variability arises, it should become the friend rather than the enemy of theorists of aging. Variability is not something that should be wished away for simplicity's sake; it should instead be actively seized to produce fresh and innovative theories of aging that do right by the complexity of our subject matter.

The fourth hallmark of contemporary aging identified by Settersten and Trauten (2009: 458) is "the big 'ifs': old age as a highly contingent period." They suggest that uncertainty today is different than it was a half century to a full century ago, particularly because basic conditions of life and death have changed so much. It has become more possible to plan since there have been decreases in mortality, morbidity, and fertility rates. However, they point out that in many parts of the world life cannot be counted on because of political and economic upheaval, war, and violence, or very poor health conditions, high rates of poverty, and high rates of mortality for people of all ages. Nevertheless, Settersten and Trauten (2009: 459) argue that old people today have far greater predictability and choice that at any time in history because of longer life and better health and improved aggregate standing compared to previous cohorts as reflected in financial and other indicators of well-being.

Settersten and Trauten (2009: 459) argue that a primary difference between old age today and in the past is its highly contingent quality. They suggest that there is a great deal of possibility in old age, but realization of its potential depends on "ifs," especially in life, health, and resources, that cannot be predicted or controlled. The ways that the "ifs" play out are related to dimensions including social class, family resources and ties, cohort, and gender. Addressing "shifting sands and mines of old age" that are conditioned by these variables, Settersten and Trauten (2009: 459) predict that social class will become the most important factor in determining aging and life course experiences and creating social cleavages. They predict that:

> …inequalities generated by social class will likely trump inequalities that stem from gender, race, and ethnicity and will yield additional power *through* these other statuses. Individuals with adequate resources early in life often accumulate resources over time, while those with fewer or no resources

stay the course at best.... This results in significant disparities in financial, social, and other resources by old age.... This chasm is likely to persist – and even grow – in the future.

According to Settersten and Trauten (2009: 459–60), in all substantive areas social class should be a central focal point. They note the current lack of attention to social class in aging scholarship and policy making. Life expectancy, physical and psychological health, family structure and relationships, social integration and engagement, personal resources, and other aspects of aging and old age are shaped by social class. Intersections between social class and race, ethnicity, and immigration status are important phenomena to consider. Furthermore, understanding the growing diversity of the aging population is about understanding differences that generate and are generated by inequality. Issues related to the shifting racial and ethnic composition of the older population include:

> What does it mean to grow old in an increasingly diverse and unequal society and to grow old as a member of one of these groups? How is diversity altering the terrain of old age and creating reverberations in periods of life before it? How might the social institutions and policies that serve old people be rearchitected in light of it? These questions demand exploration and will require (and also lead to) new theories to guide them.
>
> (Settersten and Trauten 2009: 259)

In their consideration of families as risk absorbers and risk takers, Settersten and Trauten (2009: 461) present the idea that family relationships can provide help and protection in old age but also create risks for men and women. Social policies include many assumptions about the presence and nature of family relationships that are no longer warranted, especially because of changes in marriage, divorce and remarriage rates, and other aspects of family life. New complexities, disruptions, and ambiguities in relationships have accompanied these changes and created risks, but longer lives and better health have resulted in more durable and active social relationships, a more varied mix of family and nonfamily ties, and "the ability to inhabit family and other roles in novel ways."

"Shifting sands" in the lives of older adults also include revolutions in cohort composition and experiences and consideration of cohorts past, present, and future. Settersten and Trauten (2009: 460) advise that it is important to study people belonging to cohorts in which people are not yet old in addition to cohorts such as the "baby boomers" who are new to the ranks of older adults. They also address distinctive characteristics of the baby boom generation in comparison to previous cohorts and describe implications for theory development (Settersten and Trauten 2009: 461–2):

> ...doom-and-gloom public discourse surrounding the baby boom generation has focused on how its size has strained the social institutions through which it has moved during early and middle adulthood. There is little doubt these

challenges will continue as members of the baby boom move through old age. But it is important to remember that the physical, psychological, and social statuses of boomers are extremely favorable relative to cohorts past – or at least the early cohorts of boomers. In fact one could argue that in the future there may not be another group of people who enter old age as *uniformly* well positioned as these early boomers. (The cohorts that make up the tail end of the baby boomers do not seem as advantaged as the earlier members of the generation.) Important theoretical advances will be found by probing the implications of their better positions for all aspects of aging as well as by probing their assumptions about and perspectives on old age, which will yield insights into the new and emerging models of old age for which they are striving.

Settersten and Trauten (2009: 463) suggest that the effects on later adulthood of "breakups in the gendered life course" experienced by women and men in the baby boom generation through divorce and remarriage at higher rates than in previous generations will be important to examine in theory and research. They note that:

> …it is important to explicate how the changing choices and circumstances of women earlier in life will flavor and even determine the choices and circumstances they face later in life. It is also interesting to wonder whether women's lifelong commitments to diverse and multiple roles might also make it easier for women to adjust to changes and manage hardships when they are old….
>
> Men's family relationships are especially important to watch, particularly the connections between men and children. Surprisingly, a range of social indicators reveal that men are, as a group – and contrary to public perception – becoming *less* intensely involved with and committed to children…. Divorce is particularly important to understand because it often leads to a loss or restriction of fathers' ties to children.

Settersten and Trauten (2009: 463) also emphasize that it is important for theorists and researchers to address the influence of race and ethnicity on aging experiences since trends in educational and occupational attainment, family formation, and earnings can differ dramatically for women and men, particularly in subgroups differentiated by variations in race, ethnicity, and social class. As explained by Stoller and Gibson (2000) in their approach to the life course perspective, theorists and researchers need to be mindful that differential attainments and experiences in subgroups earlier in life result in different financial, social, and psychological experiences in later adulthood.

Settersten and Trauten (2009: 468) also ask theorists, researchers, and policy makers in aging to understand the significance of the fact that most people engaging in this work are not old. They state that although everyone has had direct experiences with old people, most people studying later adulthood are younger and therefore outsiders to the people and phenomena they hope to understand. This presents challenges for theory and research because these theorists, policy makers and researchers can only assume what it is like to be old, and their assumptions affect what is done and not done with and for old people. Furthermore, Settersten and Trauten (2009: 468) suggest that knowledge about aging may have a questionable quality "especially if it is not firmly anchored in the voices and perspectives of old people who can, with great depth and texture, tell us firsthand what it is actually like."

A nexus theory for analysis of the politics of aging in diverse societies

Fernando Torres-Gil (2005: 670) developed a theoretical framework for explaining the politics of aging in diverse societies and the influence of the intersection of race, ethnicity, politics, and old age on public policy. These intersections form a nexus of aging and diversity and are important to consider because of demographic trends of societal aging, increasing diversity, immigration and migration, and potential political activism by older people. Torres-Gil (2011) believes that an emerging politics of aging that is consistent with this theoretical perspective will develop over time. He asks important questions pertaining to this subject:

> What happens to public policy when race, ethnicity, and old age are mixed together? Do age, ethnicity, and race matter in politics and public policy? As nations experience growing numbers of older persons and immigrant groups, will this scenario play out in their politics of aging? Finally, to what extent do policy makers (e.g., politicians) take into account the demands of politically active minority and immigrant elders?
>
> (Torres-Gil 2005: 670)

Torres-Gil (2005) notes that little attention has been given to the rise of minority and immigrant older adults as political interest groups, competition between older homogeneous groups and a younger diverse population, and political organizing by older and minority individuals. Despite the paucity of prior research and analysis regarding these issues, Torres-Gil has succeeded in developing a useful framework for analysis of relationships among variables that contribute to development of public policy pertaining to older adults in ethnically diverse societies. While his analysis focuses primarily on the U.S., and he acknowledges that this reduces the applicability and generalization of his theoretical framework to nations with different forms of political systems, cultures, and histories, Torres-Gil (2005: 670) suggests that it provides useful clues and suggestions "for understanding the possibility that age, race, and diversity can complicate a politics of ageing and the public policy responses to the rise of such interest groups." The diversity of nations facing a politics of aging and diversity suggests areas for additional research and theory development.

Torres-Gil (2005; Torres-Gil and Moga 2001) developed a conceptual framework for bringing together relevant factors for understanding aging and public policy in ethnically diverse societies. According to Torres-Gil (2005), the key factors in his equation – aging, public policy, ethnicity, and diversity – are usually viewed in isolation, and this framework brings them together and adds the element of politics. The premise behind his "2000–10 framework" was his belief that 2000–10 would be a very different aging period in the U.S. compared to earlier time periods. He points out that between 1935 and 1990, entitlement programs and public benefits for older people in the U.S. expanded, and there was political activism among older adults that was accompanied by sympathetic public response (see Chapter 4 for examples). Torres-Gil (2005) suggested that in "the new aging" after 2000 there would be substantially different policy and programmatic responses by government. Political and social responses would be shaped by the aging of baby boomers and related demographic imperatives; diversity, immigration, and growth in the number of older adults belonging to ethnic and racial minority groups; and the increasing challenges of maintaining the fiscal solvency of large-scale entitlement programs. He suggested that these factors might result in "a more robust politics of aging buffeted by a nation becoming more ethnically diverse. This in turn may result in tensions and competition, as well as opportunities, as older Whites, older minorities, younger immigrant groups, and a younger population in general vie for scarce public resources in a time when age-based entitlement programs will lose public support" (Torres-Gil 2005: 472). Debates in the U.S. and European Union about the fiscal crisis and retrenchment of social welfare benefits for older adults portend this influence on the emerging politics of aging (Torres-Gil 2011).

He emphasizes that it is important to invest in young immigrant communities today so that the tax base needed to fund services for the baby boomers will be available tomorrow, and he notes that Los Angeles County has continued to prosper from diversity and remain viable economically because of the influx of Armenians, Persians, Asian Pacific Islanders, Central Americans, and Latinos (Meltzer 2009). According to Torres-Gil (Meltzer 2009), baby boomers may become the next generation of senior citizen activists since the U.S. has not prepared for increased longevity and will need an engaged citizenry to compensate for inadequate planning and the crises in finance, savings, and housing.

Torres-Gil (2005: 472) points out that an age-based politics of aging in a diverse society is not a given. This will not happen automatically even though there will be more people who are older and more minority and immigrant groups. Political action or a public policy response will depend on "a fluid set of relationships that specify how various factors might influence each other" (Torres-Gil 2005: 673). Figure 8.1 explains factors and relationships in Torres-Gil's topical equation and demonstrates that potential fluid influences include diversity (D), aging (A), politics (PO), public policy (PP), and politics of aging (PoA). Likewise, Torres-Gil's framework asks us to consider the extent to which politics and public policy have caused older and more diverse groups to become interested in politics of aging. This model suggests that a politics of aging can result from increased diversity within an aging population and/or be a result of attempts to reform public benefits that impact older and diverse populations.

Causal relationships

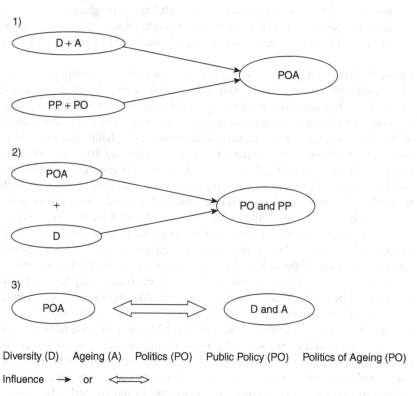

Figure 8.1 Key factors in the topical equation and the fluid influences that may result.

Source: *Torres-Gil, F.* (2005) "Ageing and public policy in ethnically diverse societies," in M. Johnson (ed.) *The Cambridge Handbook of Age and Ageing.* Reprinted with the permission of Cambridge University Press.

Torres-Gil (2005) believes that in the U.S. a politics of aging that includes diversity has resulted from the increase in minority, racial, and immigrant groups with substantial numbers of older adults. Organizations representing African American, American Indian, Asian and Pacific Islander, and Hispanic elders exist. Adults age 65 and over in ethnic and racial minority groups are more likely to vote than younger cohorts. Furthermore, minority groups, particularly Hispanics and Asian and Pacific Islanders, are becoming the numerical majority in some regions, especially in the Southwestern U.S., increasing their political power. Torres-Gil (2005) affirms that African Americans, Asians, and Hispanics are increasingly exercising political influence in domestic areas including education, social welfare, and healthcare, and influencing foreign policy areas including immigration relations with Mexico, South Africa, and China. He (2005: 674) asks:

What would happen if these groups were to take an interest in ageing-related policies such as potential reforms of entitlement programs (e.g., Social Security, Medicare)? What electoral role might these voters play? To what extent will minority elders become a significant force in a politics of ageing?

Although Torres-Gil (2005: 674) believes that the U.S. has a political system in which public policies are increasingly influenced by ethnically diverse and older populations, the model illustrated in Figure 8.1 may not be applicable to parts of the world with different political systems. A systematic analysis of applicability of this theory to other nations requires determination of whether there are indications that organizing by older people is occurring in the country under consideration and whether the political systems and public policies are susceptible to a politics of aging. Furthermore, does the society have aspects of diversity in the areas of race, culture, ethnicity, and immigration that could intersect with aging?

Torres-Gil (2005) points out that most nations do not have the open and pluralistic democratic political system that exists in the U.S. and provides a form of civic culture that facilitates interest group organizing by all interested constituents. Replication of the U.S. politics of aging may be limited by existence of a more top-down model of government in many countries and by the reality that age may not be the dominant variable in how an older person exercises political choice. Furthermore, many factors affect old age policy issues in addition to actions taken by older people (Torres-Gil 205: 674). Despite these realities, older people in some nations are acquiring age consciousness and organizing around concerns related to their experiences as older adults. For example, China has been confronted with rebellious activities by Chinese retirees angry about political corruption and unpaid or disappearing pensions. In the Netherlands, pensioners have resisted dilution of their subsidies, and age-based political parties have developed. Aging-based political organizations have developed in Australia, Canada, Japan, and Europe. Torres-Gil (2005: 675) suggests that:

> we are witnessing the potential emergence of varied forms of a politics of ageing in different parts of the world. And, with the continued graying of many of these nations, the high costs of social welfare programs for older persons, and declining fertility levels, we may find that old age matters in their politics, especially where fundamental changes to pensions and healthcare programs adversely affect older persons.

Torres-Gil (2005) contrasts aging policy development in the U.S. and South Korea, a more homogeneous country with a different history of political systems and an incipient politics of aging. South Korea has a traditional Confucian culture with an overriding value of filial piety that includes forms of affection, repayment, respect, and responsibility toward older adults. The nation is aging at the same time as it is becoming more Westernized, and the percentage of older people in South Korea's population is projected to increase from 3.2 percent in

1960 to over 19 percent in 2030. The rapid aging of the population is creating tensions within traditional family relationships. Torres-Gil (2005: 677) continues:

> One survey shows that about two-thirds of Korean adults in their 20s to 50s would prefer to live independently of their children when they are old (Jung-Ki and Torres-Gil, 2000). In addition, the Korean government has embarked on a program to develop long term care facilities, retirement pensions, and medical and social programs for the elderly. Where these trends may eventually lead – a more Western model of individualism, ageism, isolation of elders, or maintenance of the traditional practice of filial piety – is uncertain.
>
> On the surface, Korea may appear removed from the historical, cultural, economic, and political conditions that gave rise to a politics of ageing in the United States. But on closer examination, some of those preconditions may be unfolding in Korean society.

Torres-Gil (2005: 677) has theorized that specific preconditions are necessary for a society to have a basis for a politics of aging similar to that of the U.S. The preconditions are:

1. longevity and the rise of multigenerational families;
2. a capitalist, free-market environment, the pressures of modernization, and a competitive global economy;
3. the rise of individualism, opportunity (e.g., education, professional advancement), and a move towards nuclear family households;
4. elder dissatisfaction with changes in the family and society and growing isolation from family and community;
5. an open, pluralistic democracy with an unfettered media;
6. interest group politics and the rise of advocacy and constituent-based organizations;
7. the presence of older individuals serving as advocates and spokespersons for their age cohort;
8. the adoption of Western systems of categorical programs for the elderly; and
9. the prevalence of a youth-oriented culture and of ageism.

According to Torres-Gil (2005: 678), South Korean society has met the preconditions of longevity and multigenerational families; capitalism, modernization, and a competitive global economy; movement toward individualism and nuclear family households; and elder dissatisfaction with changes in family and society and growing isolation from family and community. He believes that Korean society is on the verge of a growing youth-oriented society and signs of reluctance to care for older relatives within family households (described by Torres-Gil as ageism); development of Western systems of categorical programs; and pluralistic democracy. Development of interest group politics and advocacy and constituent-based organizations, as well as older people who serve as advocates and spokespeople for their cohort, remain as the final preconditions to be achieved for the politics of aging described in Torres-Gil's theoretical perspective.

Torres-Gil (2005: 678) asserts that in his nexus model the element of diversity must be present. In this model, diversity refers to the

> differences within a population and is best exemplified where the majority population is relatively homogeneous and older but must account for different cultures, races, and ethnicities in its midst that are younger. This is otherwise known as an 'age-race stratified' society…. Differences in fertility rates play a key role in an age-race stratified society.
>
> (Torres-Gil 2005: 678–9)

Diversity is apparent in the U.S. where the replacement ratio of the White non-Hispanic population is lower than the rate for the Asian, Black, and Hispanic populations. Likewise, the potential for an age-race stratified society is apparent in Western European countries, and in Denmark, France, and Germany fertility rates in the native population have been lower than rates for Arab, Algerian, and Turkish guest workers. In Israel, the older population is primarily of European origin; in contrast, there is more diversity in the younger population because of the declining birth rate and substantial immigration from African and Middle Eastern nations (Torres-Gil 2005: 679).

Torres-Gil (2005: 679–80) has outlined the basis for public policy in an aging and ethnically diverse society:

> While we may not yet have clarity about the direction and evolution of ageing and public policy in ethnically diverse societies, the importance and relevance of this topical trend grows. A globalized world can no longer view its demographic changes in isolation from other countries. Technological flexibility in communication (Internet), common market arrangements (e.g., North and South America, Asia), trade and economic dispersion, as well as labor and workforce mobility mean that no nation is immune from the demographic pressures facing much of the world. In due course, older and developed nations (e.g. the First World) will need the youthful populations of the Third World. Maintaining expensive social programs with a declining labor and tax base will require fundamentally difficult decisions about reductions in public benefits or promoting the growth of younger immigrant and minority populations. And the aspirations of disenfranchised minorities and immigrant groups living longer will increase demands and expectations for the 'good life' enjoyed by retirees in affluent nations. What is certain is that diversity will become a crucial variable in the evolution of a politics of ageing in much of the world, and, in turn, politics and public policy will influence a politics of ageing and be influenced by it. Further research and monitoring of demographic trends, politics, government responses, and immigration may reveal possibilities of this occurring.

Cross-cultural analysis of theories, policies, and realities of assistance for older adults in the welfare state

Swedish gerontologist Mats Thorslund and U.S. gerontologist Merril Silverstein (2009) have developed a theoretical framework for analysis and prediction of global trends in public policies addressing aging under contemporary pressures of globalization. They begin their discussion with the observation that most Western societies have retrenched social welfare programs in efforts to shift responsibility for assistance to older people from governments to individuals and families.

According to Thorslund and Silverstein (2009: 630), nations labeled welfare states, those with "the most universal, generous, and egalitarian systems of care and support to their older citizens…are said to be at the greatest risk of crisis." These theorists (2009: 630) have explored the welfare state as a sociocultural ideal and "an institution tied historically to the material conditions that gave rise to it and sustains it," and they believe that the welfare state is being reevaluated primarily because "the economic, political, and social conditions that seeded its growth have changed. External constraints on the welfare state rising from global market integration and reduced public budgets have opened up an internal contradiction between the political and moral economies that underlie the welfare state." They assert that the contradiction is especially apparent in policies pertaining to the older population in Scandinavian countries, where the idealized form of welfare state development in support and care of older people has existed (Thorslund and Silverstein 2009).

Thorslund and Silverstein (2009: 630) present a paradigm that includes three approaches for allocation of formal services to dependent older persons in more developed nations, drawing on Esping-Andersen's (1990, 1999) typology. The groupings are:

(a) *social democratic welfare states* in which all citizens are incorporated under a single universal insurance system (such as those found in the Scandinavian countries);

(b) *liberal welfare states*, where assistance is means tested and modest social insurance plans dominate (such as those found in Australia, Canada, and the United States); and the

(c) *conservative welfare states* where the state will only intervene when the family's resources are exhausted (such as Austria, France, and Germany).

In most developing nations, residual policies exist that leave the majority of care responsibilities to families (Thorslund and Silverstein 2009).

According to Thorslund and Silverstein (2009: 630), theories "locate the welfare state as an evolutionary end product of societal development and modernization." There have been three distinct historical phases in development of the welfare state, and each phase has corresponded with a particular institutional response to aging populations (Phillipson 2003; Thorslund and Silverstein 2009).

The welfare state began in the 1950s, and as it rapidly expanded through the mid-1970s, state-supported pensions for older people increased and home help services and residential care became readily available. Thorslund and Silverstein (2009: 630) describe early development of the welfare state as fueled "by economic expansion, close to full employment rates, and the near sanctification of the intergenerational contract, this period is often referred to as the 'golden age' of the welfare state." They describe the second phase, from the late 1970s through the 1990s, as "characterized by skepticism and even hostility toward the welfare state fueled by growing economic instability, declining real wages, and loss of faith in the viability of institutions supporting older people" (Thorslund and Silverstein 2009: 630). The decade of 2000–10 was the beginning of the third phase, a period described by Thorslund and Silverstein (2009: 631) as:

> shaped by the expansion of global trade, the near worship of free markets, and the perceived competitive advantage of having a smaller public sector. In this new economic environment, population aging – specifically the demands that an aging population places on the public sector – has become increasingly considered an obstacle to global competitiveness.

Thorslund and Silverstein (2009: 631) cite Razin and Sadka's (2005) especially gloomy scenario projecting that the old age dependency ratio in European Union nations will experience an increase in the range 35 percent to 66 percent between 2000 and 2050 due to population aging. Razin and Sadka (2005) suggest that tax increases of up to 33 percent or debt financing would be required to pay the obligations owed to older citizens. They suggest that both of these alternatives would slow the economic growth of European nations.

Thorslund and Silverstein (2009: 631) suggest that there are major differences in challenges of population aging that face European nations:

> For the developed welfare states of Scandinavia, the challenge is to ensure that existing systems for long-term care and pensions can withstand the demands exerted by increasing needs and numbers (both in absolute terms but especially in relative terms) of elderly persons in the population. In the less developed welfare states (e.g., Italy, Spain, and Greece), the challenge will more be to develop new systems and finding the resources necessary to fund them.

There are strong differences among Western European countries in preferences for state or family support for frail elders, ranging from overwhelming support for public care in Norway to a strong preference in Spain for a mix of public and family care (Thorslund and Silverstein 2009).

Sweden in comparative context

Sweden, a monarchy with a parliamentary form of government and a population of 9 million people, provides an important location for Thorsland and Silverstein's reevaluation of a social democratic welfare state in which there has been strong public support for extensive public funding of health and social services since the 1950s. The three independent government levels are the national government, county councils, and municipalities. According to the World Health Organization (Glenngård et al. 2005):

> Quality health care for all is a cornerstone of the Swedish welfare state. The 1982 Health and Medical Services Act not only incorporates equal access to services on the basis of need, it also emphasizes a vision of equal health for all. Three basic principles are intended to apply to health and medical care in Sweden. The principle of 'human dignity' means that all human beings have an equal entitlement to dignity, and should have the same rights, regardless of their status in the community. The principle of 'need and solidarity' means that those in greatest need take precedence in medical care. The principle of 'cost-effectiveness' means that when a choice has to be made from different health care options, there should be a reasonable relationship between the costs and the effects, measured in terms of improved health and improved quality of life.

Thorslund and Silverstein (2009: 633) suggest that development of Swedish welfare state exceptionalism can be attributed to the confluence of the following conditions after World War II:

(a) rapid economic growth enabled by a relatively intact infrastructure and male labor force after the war and access to rich natural resources;

(b) high levels of public trust in state institutions and their representatives earned by a government with little corruption and a good degree of transparency;

(c) a small and homogeneous population that minimized internal conflict over resource allocation; and

(d) a strong state church that could provide institutional leverage for welfare state policies.

They note that some of these conditions have changed. There is no longer a state-sanctioned church, a change that reflects increasing secularization and greater ethnic and religious heterogeneity as a result of a generous immigration policy. Also, the Social Democrats were able to establish generous social policy during the booming economy of the 1950s, but in weaker economic times difficult decisions have been required pertaining to budget reductions and elimination of services. However, there continues to be broad public support for the Social Democratic political party and liberal social welfare policies ensuring availability of extensive government services to all across the lifespan (Arvidsson 2011; Lilekvist 2011; Stayton 2011a).

In 2011, the national income tax rate in Sweden was 25 percent, and the average total income tax rate was 57 percent (Tax Rates CC 2011). The mean municipal tax rate was 20.73 percent, and the county council mean rate was 10.82 percent (Statistics Sweden 2011). The value added tax (VAT) for goods and services is 25 percent of assessed value except for certain items that are tax exempt or taxed at 6 percent or 12 percent (Tax Rates CC 2011). The Swedish government has continued to provide a pension to all residents, and people are entitled to receive the pension at age 60 regardless of employment status (Stayton 2011b). The amount is based on the number of years employed and amount of salary, and some people also receive pensions from unions and pension organizations. There is some public concern about the possibility of reductions in the amounts paid in government pensions, and there is also discussion about the idea of a policy change that would allow continued employment past the current retirement ages of 65 and 67 (Stayton 2011b). Most workers are in unions, but in recent years privatization has given people more options for employment in non-union work settings (Lilekvist 2011).

The timeline for development of public care for older adults in Sweden began after World War II with provision of institutional care. During the 1950s, municipalities began to provide in-home support to dependent older adults, and in 1956 the policy of legal obligation of children to care for their parents was abolished. The option of remaining at home and receiving public help became a goal for assistance to older adults. The services provided at home were primarily domestic services such as cooking, cleaning and laundry, and people with more extensive service needs received institutional care. State subsidies were introduced to the municipalities in Sweden in the mid-1960s, and service use increased rapidly. Recipients paid only a small fraction of the cost of home help, and by the late 1970s, almost 25 percent of retired Swedes received assistance at some time during the year. This coincided with the developing Swedish economy and general growth of public welfare services during the 1960s and 1970s. At the same time, more middle-aged women were able to enter the labor market rather than care for dependent parents at home. By the mid-1980s, demand for home help services exceeded what the public system could provide, and stricter needs assessments led to the average service recipient being a person with more extensive health problems. Service demands have grown as the proportion of the population that is age 80 and older has increased to exceed 5 percent of the population (Thorslund and Silverstein 2009).

Public services for older people are divided into provision of health care through county councils and elder care provided by municipalities. This structure resulted from public criticism of the organization of care and establishment of a new elder care policy in 1992. In addition to providing home help services, municipalities were given responsibility for nursing home care for patients who could not go directly home upon hospital discharge. Weakening economic growth in the 1990s resulted in additional restructuring of long-term care that increased pressure on public providers of municipal elder care. Home help services were targeted to the most frail and dependent elderly with personal care needs; in service provision to married couples, the spouse was often the only caregiver and needed to make informal arrangements for assistance. While municipalities began to contract services to nonpublic providers, commercial and volunteer alternatives to out-of-pocket payments continue to be almost nonexistent (Thorslund and Silverstein 2009).

Over 10 percent of the older adults in Denmark, Finland, Norway, and Sweden received home help in the early 1990s, and this was a higher rate than other European nations and more than twice the rate in the U.S. However, Sweden reduced the rate to 8 percent during the 1990s although at 6.6 hours per week it provided greater intensity of care than the other Scandinavian countries. This reflected a strategy to target the older adults most in need and provide adequate assistance to keep frail older people in their homes for as long as possible. However, this strategy did not meet the needs of people with more moderate needs who would find assistance helpful (Thorslund and Silverstein 2009: 631–2).

The Swedish government continues to adhere to the general principle that social care and health care for older people are primarily public sector tasks and provides a broad range of services including health care and long-term care, supervision of county administrative boards focusing on social service issues by the National Board of Health and Welfare, provision of grants for housing adaptation so that elderly people with disabilities can continue to live at home, and provide home care and adult day care services (Regeringskansliet 2010). Although government is the primary provider of social and health care for older people and this role is expected by the public (Arvidsson 2011; Garcia-Quinteros 2011; Lilekvist 2011; Peju 2011), social services are also provided by religious and secular nongovernmental organizations (NGOs). In the city of Eskilstuna, priests and deacons in the parishes of the Swedish Lutheran Church, the former state church, provide extensive social service assistance to older adults and their families (Arvidsson 2011; Garcia-Quinteros 2011; Peju 2011; Granberg 2011; Stayton 2011a). In addition to assistance that is provided to Swedish older adults and their families, help is provided to people from very diverse cultural backgrounds by parish staff who speak a total of 17 languages, and staff members are sensitive to the influence of culture and history on the lives of older people and the ways that these differences influence family relationships and expectations of old age (Arvidsson 2011; Garcia-Quinteros 2011; Granberg 2000; Peju 2000; Stayton 2000a). Eskilstuna is an industrial city where opportunities for employment have historically been plentiful and resettlement by refugees encouraged, and therefore the communities served by the parish include people from very diverse nations, including Chile, Iran, Iraq, Hungary, Egypt, and Somalia (Arvidsson 2011). The parish provides substantial assistance to Finnish older adults, many of whom worked in the steel mills and formed their own Finnish community, but as their friends and relatives die they need meeting places in and out of church where Finnish is spoken (Peju 2011).

Additional nongovernmental resources in Eskilstuna include services provided by the Salvation Army, the "Caritas" program of the Roman Catholic Church, and a center where services are available through NGOs such as the Red Cross to assist families of older adults (Garcia-Quinteros 2011; Peju 2011; Stayton 2011b), and there are also voluntary organizations that were established by community residents when a need developed (Arvidsson 2011). For example, in Eskilstuna there is an organization initiated by community residents who identified the need for services for people coping with kidney diseases. There are many private doctors and a few private hospitals, including some operated by Roman Catholic orders (Stayton 2011b). There is also a history in Sweden of older people organizing for advocacy on their own behalf, including activism by members of the National Organization of Pensioners (PRO) in resistance to enemies and injustices identified as forces of the past (Jonson 2005), and more recent activism because there are older people who believe that political parties, church, and society in general are pushing them out (Arvidsson 2011; Stayton 2011a).

A report by the World Health Organization Regional Office for Europe (Glenngård et al. 2005) on behalf of the European Observatory on Health Systems and Policies documents that Sweden has one of the world's oldest populations, with over 17 percent of the population at least age 65 and 5.2 percent at least age 85. Sweden has had negative natural population growth since the late 1990s but has experienced population growth due to positive net migration flow. Consistent with international trends noted by Settersten and Trauten and Torres-Gil, the WHO report indicates that

> ageing of Swedish society has important social and political implications, as fewer persons of productive age are available to provide financial support for the increasing demands being placed on the health care system. It is estimated that by the year 2050, more than 23% of the population will be at least 65 years old and 8.4% will be at least age 80 years old.
>
> (Statistics Sweden 2004, in Glenngård et al. 2005: 3–4)

Offering a comparative perspective, Thorslund and Silverstein (2009: 631) assert that:

> Swedish policies ... are designed to reduce the burden placed on families, especially women, by their elder care responsibilities. Recent evidence demonstrates that the Swedish model is effective in meeting the needs of elders. Impaired elders in the United States are more likely to have unmet needs compared to similarly impaired elders in Sweden, and this disparity is almost completely explained by the lower use of formal services in the United States (Shea et al., 2003). Further, research suggests that compared to the United States the formal service sector of Sweden better targets institutional care at more vulnerable elders, suggesting that both greater coverage *and* greater efficiencies are achieved by the welfare state
>
> (Davey et al., 2005).

Thorslund and Silverstein (2009: 634) theorize:

> Even though the economic situation in Sweden has recovered from the recession in the 1990s, a simple thought experiment would lead to the conclusion that if Sweden had not chosen as it did in the 1950s and 1960s to develop

a welfare state regime, it would unlikely have done so today. What this means for more conservative welfare states is that the establishment of a Scandinavian-style welfare state is highly unlikely. If the Scandinavian ideal is out of step with the current trend toward smaller and more conservative governments in Europe and North America (and most recently in Sweden itself), what, then, is the future of the welfare state in the very nations that brought it into being as a third way between communism and capitalism?...

The system of old-age support and care in Sweden embodies principles of universalism in allocating benefits and services to the elderly with the goal that socioeconomic differentials should be minimized and collectivization of risk maximized (Daatland, 1997; Thorslund, 1991).

In general, Scandinavian social welfare systems provide cradle-to-grave protections against economic and social needs caused by unemployment, poor health, retirement, and family formation with every citizen in principle having equal access to benefits. To simplify a bit, the welfare state rests on two pillars: a political economy in which economic growth and relatively high taxes allowed its establishment, expansion, and sustenance and a moral economy that legitimates the universalistic and redistributive principles under which it sets policies.

Thorsland and Silverstein (2009: 634) identify primary issues to consider in differentiating between systems. They identify the tension between moral and political economies in which more egalitarian moral values are in conflict with pressures experienced by policymakers to apply market principles, privatization, in designing more restrictive social welfare programs. They also raise questions about collective obligations to older people and rights of older people to health and supportive services. In the U.S., the issue of public and private risk plays a major role in policy debates about income security and health care for older people, and trends toward individualization of risk permeate U.S. social institutions.

Thorslund and Silverstein (2009: 635) assert that:

> ...moral economy reflects the underlying values and preferences in each national population and preferences in each national population of the 'good' society – what is desirable even if not achievable. These valuations include the relationship between private and public responsibility for older adults, the role of women in the labor market and in family roles, the amount of autonomy and residential independence that care systems provide older persons, and the role of the private and voluntary sector in the care mix....

Discussions among policymakers in developed welfare states tend to follow narrow technocratic lines such as how to get the most efficiency out of existing systems. The welfare state is entrenched bureaucratically and politically, making change difficult, but it is also ideologically ingrained in the public mind. The welfare state remains popular in Nordic countries, even though confidence in it is waning. Institutional inertia guarantees that change when it comes will be incremental. In addition, the welfare state has raised expectations in the population based on what an earlier generation of adults received, making severe cutbacks politically unpopular in many circles. Given the global and demographic forces at work, modifications to the welfare state are inevitable. Acceptance of the policy changes in the offing may hinge on whether citizens perceive them as retrenchment or reconstruction of the social welfare enterprise (Quadagno & Street, 2006).

Thorslund and Silverstein (2009: 638) conclude that, in the end, "demography is not destiny for the welfare state but may require a detour that is compatible with the national character on which it is based."

Advocacy for global policies for the well-being of older people

Many organizations are addressing challenges experienced by older adults and their families and responding to issues reflected in predictions of theorists and researchers addressing demographic, economic, political, and social changes and their potential for affecting the lives of older people negatively. The United Nations, World Health Organization, The Global Alliance for the Rights of Older People, and national, regional, and local public agencies and nongovernmental organizations (NGOs) are addressing the effects of globalization with aggressive initiatives by and on behalf of older people. Members of The Global Alliance are organizations addressing a broad range of issues related to aging: International Network for the Prevention of Elder Abuse (INPEA), International Longevity Centre (ILC), Global Alliance, International Federation on Ageing (IFA), International Association of Homes and Services for the Aged (IAHSA), International Association of Gerontology and Geriatrics (IAGG), HelpAge International, Global Action on Ageing (GAA), Age UK, and AARP. In addition, major global initiatives include the United Nations (UN) *Political Declaration and Madrid International Plan of Action on Ageing* adopted in 2002 and related subsequent actions, including the Open-ended Working Group on Ageing for the Purpose of Strengthening the Protection of the Human Rights of Older Persons established by the UN General Assembly in 2010. A major World Health Organization (WHO) initiative established in 2006 is the Age-friendly Cities Programme. These initiatives are driven by values of human rights and social justice and include planning and programs to improve the well being of older people throughout the world.

United Nations *Political Declaration and Madrid International Plan of Action on Ageing*

The *Political Declaration and Madrid International Plan of Action on Ageing* was adopted at the UN Second World Assembly on Ageing in Madrid, Spain, in 2002, and acknowledges common features of aging and the diversity of aging experiences throughout the world. The Assembly was attended by representatives from 158 nations, and the overarching goal of their political declaration and plan is to:

> ...ensure that persons everywhere are able to age with security and dignity and to continue to participate in their societies as citizens with full rights. While recognizing that the foundation for a healthy and enriching old age is laid early in life, the plan is intended to be a practical tool to assist policy makers to focus on the key priorities associated with individual and population ageing. The common features of the nature of ageing and the challenges it presents are acknowledged and specific recommendations are designed to be adapted to the great diversity of circumstances that are taking place in various regions, as well as the interdependence of all countries in a globalizing world.
>
> (UN 2002c: 17)

The declaration and plan followed previous commitments to foster a society for all ages by heads of state and governments at major UN conferences and summits and follow up processes, the UN Millennium Declaration, the International Plan of Action on Ageing endorsed by the UN General Assembly in 1982, and the UN Principles for Older Persons adopted by the General Assembly in 2001. In addition to work on implementation of the Madrid Plan, ongoing advocacy continues for a UN Convention on the Rights of Older Persons that would strengthen the commitments to the rights of older people that exist in the Madrid Plan.

The following central themes run through the International Plan of Action and are linked to specific goals, objectives, and commitments:

(a) The full realization of all human rights and fundamental freedoms of all older persons;

(b) The achievement of secure ageing, which involves reaffirming the goal of eradicating poverty in old age and building on the United Nations Principles for Older Persons;

(c) Empowerment of older persons to fully and effectively participate in the economic, political and social lives of their societies, including through income-generating and voluntary work;

(d) Provision of opportunities for individual development, self-fulfillment and well-being throughout life as well as in late life, through, for example, access to lifelong learning and participation in the community while recognizing that older persons are not one homogeneous group;

(e) Ensuring the full enjoyment of economic, social, and cultural rights, and civil and political rights of persons and the elimination of all forms of violence and discrimination against older persons;

(f) Commitment to gender equality among older persons through, interalia, elimination of gender-based discrimination;

(g) Recognition of the crucial importance of families, intergenerational interdependence, solidarity and reciprocity for social development;

(h) Provision of health care, support and social protection for older persons, including preventive and rehabilitative health care;

(i) Facilitating partnership between all levels of government, civil society, the private sector and older persons themselves in translating the International Plan of Action into practical action;

(j) Harnessing of scientific research and expertise and realizing the potential of technology to focus on, inter alia, the individual, social and health implications of ageing, in particular in developing countries;

(k) Recognition of the situation of ageing indigenous persons, their unique circumstances and the need to seek means to give them an effective voice in decisions directly affecting them.

(UN 2002c: 17–18)

The 19 Articles of the Political Declaration affirm the commitment of the government representatives at the Second World Assembly on Aging to respond to opportunities and challenges of population aging and promote development of a society for all ages. They affirm commitment to actions at all levels in the priority areas of older persons and development, health and well-being into old age, and ensuring and enabling supportive environments, and acknowledge the demographic transformation that challenges societies to promote increased opportunities, especially for full participation of older people in all aspects of life. The Articles reaffirm the previous UN commitments related to aging that provided guidance related to independence, participation, care, self-fulfillment and dignity and emphasize the necessity of international cooperation. Article 5 states the intentions of the Madrid International Plan:

We reaffirm the commitment to spare no effort to promote democracy, strengthen the rule of law and promote gender equality, as well as to promote and protect human rights and fundamental freedoms, including the right to development. We commit ourselves to eliminating all forms of discrimination, including age discrimination. We also recognize that persons, as they age, should enjoy a life of fulfillment, health, security and active participation in the economic, social, cultural and political life of their societies. We are determined to enhance the recognition of the dignity of older persons and to eliminate all forms of neglect, abuse, and violence.

(UN 2002c: 9–12)

In Articles 6 and 7 of the Political Declaration, the signers acknowledged the global opportunities and challenges:

The modern world has unprecedented wealth of technological capacity and has presented extraordinary opportunities: to empower men and women to reach old age in better health and with more fully realized well-being; to seek the full inclusion and participation of older persons in societies; to enable older persons to contribute more effectively to their communities and to the development of their societies; and to steadily improve care and support for older persons as they need it. We recognize that concerted action is required to transform the opportunities and the quality of life for men and women as they age and to ensure the sustainability of their support systems, thus building the foundation for a society for all ages. When ageing is embraced as an achievement, the reliance on human skills, experiences, and resources of the higher age groups is naturally recognized as an asset in the growth of mature, fully integrated, humane societies...

At the same time, considerable obstacles to further integration and full participation in the global economy remain for developing countries, in particular the least developed countries, as well as for some countries with economies in transition. Unless the benefits of social and economic development are extended to all countries, a growing number of people, particularly older persons in all countries and even entire regions, will remain marginalized from the global economy. For this reason, we recognize the importance of placing ageing on development agendas, as well as strategies for the eradication of poverty and in seeking to achieve full participation in the global economy of all developing nations.

(UN 2002c: 10)

The Articles also describe commitment to incorporate aging into social and economic strategies, policies, and action with the understanding that specific policies will vary because of differences in national conditions. There is recognition of the need to mainstream a gender perspective into all policies and programs, as well as acknowledgment of the importance of addressing the need for leadership by older people in the work toward future development. Coordination among governmental agencies and NGOs, provision of social services and universal access to physical and mental health services, promotion of healthy lifestyles and supportive environments, and accessibility and empowerment of older people for full participation in all aspects of society is specified. Caregiving issues are addressed: the role of older people as caregivers, the roles of diverse care providers for older adults, and the importance of mutually responsive relationships between generations. Governments are expected to assume primary responsibility for leadership on aging matters and implementation of the Madrid International Plan of Action on Ageing, but it was understood that implementation would also require partnership and involvement of professional organizations; corporations; workers and workers' organizations; cooperatives; research, academic and other educational and religious institutions; and the media. Furthermore the UN system, including regional commissions, is expected to provide assistance to governments requesting assistance with implementation, follow up, and national monitoring of the plan. This is to be provided with respect to differences in demographic, economic, and social conditions among countries and regions.

(UN 2002c: 10–12)

In July, 2011, the UN General Assembly issued Secretary General Ban Ki-moon's report "Follow-up to the Second World Assembly on Ageing." Consistent with the *Political Declaration and Madrid International Plan on Ageing*, the report focuses on human rights of older people throughout the world and describes challenges faced by older women and men in securing their rights. It provides examples of good practices and policies that have been developed to address human rights issues including discrimination, violence and abuse, social protection, long-term care, age-specific services, participation, and access to justice and lifelong pensions. Poverty was identified as the single most pressing challenge to the welfare of older people, including the related problems of inadequate living conditions, homelessness, malnutrition, unattended chronic diseases, lack of access to safe drinking water and sanitation, unaffordable medicines and treatments, income insecurity, and additional human rights issues. The recommendations include continuation of the UN Open-ended Working Group on Ageing that was established in 2010 (UN 2011).

The Secretary General's report also recommends that member states consider enhancing their capacity for more effective data collection, statistics, and qualitative information in order to better assess the situation and rights of older people and establish adequate monitoring mechanisms for programs. It was suggested that the General Assembly consider recommending to member states that more explicit wording about the situation of older persons be incorporated into the language of existing international instruments, treaty body monitoring mechanisms, and dialogues with states, and given higher priority in consideration of reports and the agenda of their country missions. The report also advised the General Assembly that recommendations be made to member states to design and implement more effective multisectoral policies and programs pertaining to the rights of older people and consider potential benefits to governments from cooperation and support from other stakeholders including UN specialized agencies and entities, national human rights institutions, non-governmental organizations, academic entities, and statistical institutions (UN 2011).

The World Health Organization Global Age-Friendly Cities Initiative

A major project developed by WHO to promote active aging is the Age-friendly Cities Programme, an initiative to help cities prepare for the rapid aging of populations and increasing urbanization. The initiative began in 2006 when WHO brought together representatives from 33 cities in 22 nations to identify major aspects of the urban environment that support active and healthy aging. The cities included mega-cities with over 10 million inhabitants (Mexico City, Moscow, New Delhi, Rio de Janeiro, Shanghai, and Tokyo), almost mega-cities such as Istanbul, London, and New York, and regional centers, national capitals, and small cities. A publication, *Global Age-friendly Cities: A Guide* (2007), was developed based on this research and is being used in cities throughout the world for a global network of age-friendly cities. The guide identifies eight domains of city life that are believed to influence health and quality of life of older people: outdoor spaces and buildings, transportation, housing, social participation, respect and social inclusion, civic participation and employment, communication and information, and community support and health services (WHO 2007).

The role of WHO is to coordinate the Age-friendly Cities Programme, identify and disseminate best practices, develop implementation guidelines, provide technical support and training, and review progress and plans. The initiative requires clear evidence of progress in the city's original action plan during five years that include planning, implementation, and progress evaluation. If there is clear evidence of progress, cities can proceed with a subsequent phase of anticipated continual improvement for up to 5 years. Advantages of membership in the program include:

1. "Connection to a global network of ageing and civil society experts."
2. "Access to key information about the programme: latest news, best practices, events, results, challenges and new initiatives through the Age Friendly Cities Community of Practice (www.who.int/ezcollab/afc_network)."
3. "Provision of technical guidance and training throughout the AFC implementation process."
4. "Opportunities for partnerships with other cities."

(WHO 2009: 1)

In 2011, the First International Conference on Age-friendly Cities took place in Dublin, Ireland, and brought together leaders and senior managers from members of the Global Network, senior managers of municipal authorities, CEOs interested in or already involved in an Age-friendly City initiative, civil society organizations, and senior professionals across public, private, and voluntary sectors in areas such as academia, health care, housing, research, transportation, and urban planning. The Network process allows for diversity of cities across the world and takes into account each city and region's financial and social circumstances (WHO 2011).

Example: the domain of "community support and health services" in the Global Age-Friendly Cities guide

Findings from the initial study are reflected in the domain of "Community Support and Health Services" in *Global Age-friendly Cities: A Guide* (2007: 66–71). Primary identified needs within this domain are availability of sufficient good quality, appropriate, and accessible care, and health service issues dominated the discussions in the majority of the cities. A desire expressed universally by older people in the focus groups was for basic health and income support. Participants in many cities in developing countries reported a shortage of necessary services, and services were described as poorly distributed in other cities in developing countries. The largest number of complaints were expressed in the most developed countries despite the fact that some of the developed countries have the greatest volume and range of health and community support services.

In most of the cities, the state or national government rather than the city decides the supply, organization, and financing of many health and social services. Local people in local establishments and community-based for-profit and voluntary groups have important roles in provision of care and support, and civil society has a role in voluntary work and financial support. Aspects of community support and health services that are within the scope of a city's influence are included in the guide.

The primary concerns identified in the domain of "Community Support and Health Services" were accessible care, a wider range of health services, aging well services, home care, residential facilities for people unable to live at home, a network of community services, need for volunteers, and consideration of older people in emergency situations, in addition to concerns about lack of cemetery space. The age-friendly community and health services checklist that was developed includes the following items for implementation in the participating cities, using the approaches that are most appropriate for each city:

Service accessibility

> Health and social services are well-distributed throughout the city, are conveniently co-located, and can be reached readily by all means of transportation.
>
> Residential care facilities, such as retirement homes and nursing homes, are located close to services and residential areas so that residents remain integrated in the larger community.
>
> Service facilities are safely constructed and are fully accessible for people with disabilities.
>
> Clear and accessible information is provided about the health and social services for older people.
>
> Delivery of individual services is coordinated and with a minimum of bureaucracy. Administrative and service personnel treat older people with respect and sensitivity.
>
> Economic barriers impeding access to health and community support services are minimal.
>
> There is adequate access to designated burial sites.

Offer of services

> An adequate range of health and community support services is offered for promoting, maintaining and restoring health.
>
> Home care services are offered that include health services, personal care and housekeeping.
>
> Health and social services offered address the needs and concerns of older people.

Service professionals have appropriate skills and training to communicate with and effectively serve older people.

Voluntary support

Volunteers of all ages are encouraged and supported to assist older people in a wide range of health and community settings.

Emergency planning and care

Emergency planning includes older people, taking into account their needs and capacities in preparing for and responding to emergencies.

(WHO 2007: 67–71)

Summary

Richard Settersten and Molly Trauten have identified emerging hallmarks of aging and "shifting sands and mines" that create opportunities and risks for older adults and are ripe for theoretical advances and empirical investigation. They consider altered terms of life, illness, and death; individualization of old age; new freedoms and risks in old age; and old age as a highly contingent period to be new and emerging hallmarks of old age. "Shifting sands" in the lives of older adults include revolutions in cohort composition and experiences and consideration of cohorts past, present, and future.

Fernando Torres-Gil's nexus theoretical framework addresses the politics of aging in societies with substantial diversity. He theorizes that intersection of race, ethnicity, politics, and old age form a nexus of aging and diversity that is important to consider because demographic trends of societal aging, increasing diversity, immigration and migration, and potential political activism by older people will contribute to an emerging politics of aging. According to Torres-Gil, in this model the element of diversity, otherwise known as an age-race stratified society, must be present. A systematic analysis of applicability of this theory to other nations requires the following: determination of whether the nation has aspects of diversity in the areas of race, culture, ethnicity, and immigration that could intersect with aging; indications that organizing by older people is occurring in the country under consideration; and whether the political systems and public policies are susceptible to a politics of aging. He provides a comparative analysis of South Korea and the United States.

Thorslund and Silverstein present a theoretical framework for analysis and prediction of global trends in public policies addressing aging under contemporary pressures of globalization and provide a comparative analysis of Sweden as a social democratic welfare state and the United States as a liberal welfare state. They observe that most Western societies have retrenched social welfare programs in efforts to shift responsibility for elder assistance from governments to individuals and families. According to Thorslund and Silverstein, nations labeled welfare states are at the greatest risk of crisis. They conclude that demography is not destiny for the welfare state but may require a detour compatible with a nation's character.

Many organizations, including the United Nations and the World Health Organization, are addressing challenges experienced by older adults and their families and responding to policy concerns reflected in predictions of theorists and researchers. This chapter concludes with discussion about global advocacy for policies for the well-being of older people and describes the United Nations *Political Declaration and Madrid International Plan of Action on Aging* and related activities and the World Health Organization Global Age-friendly Cities Initiative.

9 Conclusion
Major themes

Key concepts

1. Phenomenological, critical, feminist, life course, and gerotranscendence theories provide a broad range of perspectives to inform global development of gerontological theory, research, policy, and practice.
2. The theories offer multiple lenses through which we can view aging experiences, and all address important aspects of individuals' experiences and demonstrate ways that theory can inform knowledge in aging societies in times of enormous social change.
3. All of the theoretical perspectives and theories in this book are important resources for understanding variations in aging experiences and their etiology, their effects on individuals and societies, and development of responses to improve the well being of older people.
4. A theme of major importance is efficacy of theory for understanding diversity of aging experiences, including inequalities, and factors contributing to diverse experiences.
5. Another theme is the significance of authorship of theoretical perspectives and research and the importance of the author's self-awareness about what she or he brings to the subject.
6. Culturally competent approaches for developing new theoretical paradigms and traditions are essential, including examination of one's own values, assumptions, and attitudes.
7. Diversity of experiences of older adults includes differences between cohorts and differences within cohorts related to individual experiences, characteristics, and societal responses.
8. Structural aspects of aging experiences are an essential focus of theoretical perspectives and have very important implications for policy development.
9. A theme across theoretical perspectives is the goal of maximizing opportunities for older people to have healthy, fulfilling lives.
10. The imperative for continued development of sociological theories about aging experiences is situated within the context of challenges and opportunities presented by global demographic changes and globalization.

Introduction

The Conclusion summarizes major themes in the book, including responses in these theoretical perspectives to earlier positivistic perspectives in sociology; contributions of the theoretical perspectives to understanding and addressing diversity of aging experiences; structural components of aging experiences; implications of demographic change for individuals and societies, and theorists' desire to provide alternatives to a biomedical model that emphasizes bodily failures. The need for activism for human rights and social justice for older people; acknowledgment of the strengths of older people and the capacity and need of older people for self-advocacy; the need to maximize opportunities for older people to have healthy, fulfilling lives; the importance of theorists' self-awareness about what they bring to the subject; and suggestions for future theorizing about aging are additional themes.

Major themes in this book

This book documents that sociological theories of aging provide essential knowledge for understanding and responding to the needs of older people and their families, communities, and societies. Sociology is enriched by theories about aging, and those included in this book inform and stimulate thinking and responses to the global "agequake." Phenomenological, critical, feminist, life course, and gerotranscendence theories and examples of their application provide a broad range of perspectives to inform global development of gerontological theory, research, policy, and practice. They offer multiple lenses through which we can view aging experiences, and all address important aspects of individuals' experiences and demonstrate ways that theory can inform knowledge in aging societies in times of enormous social change. Each perspective helps us to understand relationships between older people and social systems and provides useful perspectives for formulation of new theories and strategies to create beneficial social changes.

Interpretive approaches

These perspectives provide effective responses to earlier positivistic theoretical perspectives in sociology that did not address differences in experiences of older people adequately. While there are research needs for which a quantitative approach is most appropriate, theoretical perspectives and research in this book document the importance of interpretive approaches to theory and research for understanding the lives and circumstances of older people. Sociological theorizing about aging has progressed in its understanding that interpretive approaches facilitate understanding of the lived experiences of diverse older adults. Phenomenological approaches and the approaches to understanding in gerotranscendence theory are examples of valuable interpretive approaches. Lars Tornstam and others have identified a need to shift away from a positivistic paradigmatic framework in which there is an assumption of a common and shared definition of reality.

Diversity of aging experiences

The perspectives in this book provide frameworks for understanding differences and similarities of older people and their social environments. All of the theoretical perspectives are important resources for understanding variations in aging experiences and their causes, their effects on individuals and societies, and developing responses to improve the well being of all older people. Frameworks such as Glen Elder, Jr.'s (1999) life course paradigmatic principles: historic time and place, timing in lives, linked lives, and human agency, and Matilda White Riley's life course paradigm (1994) are important in understanding variations in experiences. Jay Gubrium (2003) and other phenomenologists address the importance of understanding the ways that identities of older people are shaped by social, cultural, and material contexts and are expressed in persistence, adaptation, and change. Critical and feminist theories include approaches such as the matrix of domination model that provide essential perspectives for understanding structural relationships and their implications for different groups. Feminist theorists have created or revisioned theoretical concepts relating to patriarchy and the paradigm of domination, gendering processes in organizations, production and reproduction, family and the gendered welfare system.

A theme of major importance is use of theory for understanding diversity of aging experiences, including inequalities, and the factors contributing to diverse experiences. Attention to diversity has been included in multiple ways in this book: (1) diversity of gerontological theoretical perspectives in sociology; (2) diversity of systems and systemic levels that receive primary attention from each theoretical perspective; (3) diversity in approaches of theoretical perspectives to addressing variations in experiences in later adulthood; (4) examples of application of the perspectives to understanding the lives of older people who are diverse in their age, ethnicity, gender, nationality, race, sexual orientation, and social class; (5) discussion of theoretical perspectives addressing causes and implications of inequality in aging experiences and effects of intersecting inequalities; (6) discussion of the significance of cohort differences in experiences of older people; and (7) diversity of nationality and gender of theorists and researchers whose work is presented in this book.

Diversity of experiences of older adults includes differences between cohorts and differences within cohorts related to individual experiences, characteristics, and societal responses. In the political economy perspective, characteristics such as gender, race, and class are considered pivotal variables in aging since they predetermine a person's location in the social order (Estes 1991; Ovrebo and Minkler 1993). Stoller and Gibson (2000), in their approach to the life course perspective, alert theorists and researchers to the need to be mindful that differential attainments and experiences in subgroups earlier in life result in different financial, social, and psychological experiences in later adulthood and the need to continue to explore these realities.

Social structure and aging experiences

Structural aspects of aging experiences are an essential focus of theoretical perspectives and have very important implications for policy development. This is a major focus in critical aging theory and feminist perspectives related to the underlying theme that interest group politics and the market serve to reinforce pluralism that conceals systematic structures of domination and oppression. Structural topics in critical gerontology include criticism of positivistic knowledge and focus on strengths and diversity of old age, and this book includes critical theoretical perspectives about retirement policies in Europe and the U.S. Political economy theorist Carroll Estes (1991) has described political economy perspectives as addressing the reality that sociohistorical, political, and economic factors influence perceptions of a group, including perceptions of older adults as a problem group, and this perspective is apparent in Alan Walker's (2006, 2009) work. Thorslund and Silverstein (2009) describe the significance of the welfare state as a sociocultural ideal and theorize about implications for the lives of older people, particularly in social democratic welfare states like Sweden, within the context of economic, political, and social changes.

Some of the perspectives reflect concern about the biomedical model that focuses primarily on bodily failures, and phenomenological gerontologists regard their approaches to understanding narratives of everyday life of older people as a stark contrast to this model. Attention to metatheorizing, ordinary theorizing by older adults or reflection on one's life, is also an important aspect of gerotranscendence theory. Writing from a political economy perspective, Alan Walker addresses the strong historical connections between development of the welfare state and older adults and emphasizes the relationship between old age and the welfare state in order to explain risk-society analysis and to counterbalance the narratives of biomedical and biology of aging, lifestyle, and consumerism.

Strengths of older people

Many theoretical perspectives in this book acknowledge strengths of older people, including experience and support to their families and communities, and the importance of participation by older adults in theory and policy development. Wang's (1999) critical analysis of the "American seniors' movement," social movements by and on behalf of older persons in the United States to improve the welfare of older adults, is informed by the Foucauldian model of power/subject/ resistance and addresses social activism from a political economy perspective.

Authorship of theories and research

An additional theme is the significance of authorship of theoretical perspectives and research and the importance of the author's self-awareness about what she or he brings to the subject. Phenomenologists remind us that as authorship is obscured over time and conduct becomes legitimated by theoretical explanations and moral justifications, conduct becomes institutionalized and constraining (Longino and Powell 2009). Tornstam objects to positivistic perspectives in which the individual is regarded as an object directed by internal and external forces and the researcher defines the key concepts and what is considered "normal." Settersten and Trauten (2009) ask theorists, researchers, and policy makers in aging to understand the significance of the fact that most people engaging in this work are not old. They state that although everyone has had direct experiences with old people, most people studying later adulthood are outsiders to the people and phenomena that they hope to understand. This presents challenges for theory and research because these theorists, policy makers and researchers can only assume what it is like to be old, and these assumptions affect what is done and not done with and for older people. Furthermore, Settersten and Trauten (2009) suggest that knowledge about aging may have a questionable quality if it is not firmly anchored in the voices and perspectives of old people.

Future theorizing about aging

These theoretical perspectives offer many insights for future theorizing about aging. Culturally competent approaches for developing new theoretical paradigms and traditions are essential, including examination of one's own values, assumptions, and attitudes (Peggye Dilworth-Anderson and Monique Cohen 2009). Richard Settersten and Molly Trauten (2009) write that in the twenty-first century all of human experience appears to be in flux, and they identify emerging hallmarks of aging and "shifting sands and mines" that create opportunities and risks for older adults and are important areas for theoretical advances and research. They suggest that there are important opportunities to rethink theories of aging and have identified new and emerging hallmarks of old age. Consistent with Matilda White Riley's (1986) concept of structural lag, Settersten and Trauten (2009) identify the importance of exploring delays in changes in social institutions and policies. Dale Dannefer and Jessica A. Kelley-Moore (2009) assert that there have been advances in development of life course theory but that six challenges for life course studies remain. These include cohort analysis and the lack of attention to intracohort inequality; confounding of life course processes and change; need for attention to intercohort variation; time 1 encapsulation; confounding the relation between age and time; and expanding putative role of choice.

Maximizing opportunities for healthy, fulfilling lives

A theme across theoretical perspectives is the goal of maximizing opportunities for older people to have healthy, fulfilling lives. Gerotranscendence theory presents a positive shift to a more cosmic and transcendent view compared to a materialistic and rational view, and gerotranscendence involves continued development throughout life (Tornstam 2005). Consistent with this perspective, Sherman (2010) suggests that a developmental shift toward contemplation involves movement from an orientation toward "being" rather than "doing" that is not regressive. However, the performance orientation of Western societies is not conducive to achieving this developmental shift in later adulthood. From a feminist perspective, Allen and Walker (2009) argue that authorship of one's own narratives is especially important for people with subjugated histories so that they are not written by others, that continued subordination of women, older adults, and people belonging to racial and ethnic minority groups is more likely if group narratives and history are lost. The goals of the United Nations Madrid Plan of Action and the World Health Organization's Age-friendly Cities global initiative are oriented toward continued participation by older people in family, community, workplace, and religious and political life.

Content in this book informs our thinking about human rights and social justice issues in the lives of older people and can inform advocacy efforts. Feminist theorists Calasanti and Zajicek (1993) argue that the challenge to state-based patriarchal dominance depends on women's political agency to develop understanding of policies perpetuating gender inequalities. Critical theory supports the idea that history and social context influence the forms of expression of resistance, and Frank T.Y. Wang (1999) views patterns of resistance as culturally dependent. He suggests that in a liberal democratic capitalist society like the U.S., formation of organized special interest groups such as the Gray Panthers for engagement in the political process is a normative and socially accepted approach to resistance, but groups such as immigrant elders are less likely to have the power to access this hierarchically distributed form of resistance. Likewise, in societies without histories of civil participation and organizing it is more difficult to organize for change, and Wang provides the example of suicide among older Chinese women as an alternative form of resistance. Fernando Torres-Gil's (2005) theoretical framework that clarifies the politics of aging in diverse societies and the influence of the intersection of race, ethnicity, politics, and old age on public policy when there is a nexus of aging and diversity is an important contribution to understanding implications of intersecting variables. These intersections are important to consider because of the demographic trends of societal aging, increasing diversity, immigration and migration, and potential political activism by older people. Torres-Gil (2011) believes that an emerging politics of aging that is consistent with this theoretical perspective will develop over time. The diversity of nations facing a politics of aging and diversity suggest areas for additional research and theory development.

Theory development within the context of global demographic changes and globalization

The imperative for continued development of sociological theories about aging experiences is situated within the context of challenges and opportunities presented by global demographic changes and globalization. Theorists need to continue to provide insights into these changes and their implications for individuals, families, communities, and societies, and people addressing effects of changes need to avail themselves of knowledge from theoretical perspectives. As indicated in Chapter 1, evidence presented at the United Nations Second World Assembly on Ageing in Madrid in 2002 predicted that effects of global aging will be experienced in areas including economic growth; savings, investment and consumption; labor markets; pensions; taxation and transfers of wealth, property and care from one generation to another; health and health care; family composition and living arrangements; housing and migration; and political activism by and on behalf of older people. The effects of these and other changes are experienced every day by older people throughout the world and need to be addressed by approaches that maximize opportunities for well being.

Summary

The theoretical perspectives and theories in this book are important resources for understanding variations in aging experiences and the effects of gerontological diversity on individuals and societies. This chapter summarizes major themes in the book, including the significance of authorship of theoretical perspectives and research and the need for culturally competent approaches for developing new theoretical paradigms and traditions. Additional themes include the goal of maximizing opportunities for older people to have healthy, fulfilling lives, and acknowledgment of the strengths of older people and the capacity and need of older people for self-advocacy. The imperative for continued development of sociological theories about aging experiences is situated within the context of challenges and opportunities presented by global demographic changes and globalization. Structural aspects of aging experiences are identified as an essential focus of theoretical perspectives and have important implications for policy development.

Bibliography

Abrams, K. (1991) "Hearing the call of stories," *California Law Review*, 79: 971.

—— (1993) "Unity, narrative and law," in A. Serat and S.S. Sibley (eds) *Studies in Law, Politics and Society*, Greenwich, CT: JAI Press.

Abu-Lughod, J. (1993) *Writing Women's Worlds*, Berkeley: University of California Press.

Achenbaum, W.A. (2005) "Ageing and changing: international historical perspectives on ageing," in M.L. Johnson (ed.) *The Cambridge Handbook of Age and Ageing*, Cambridge, U.K.: Cambridge University Press.

Acker, J. (1988) "Class, Gender, and the Relations of Distribution," *Signs*, 13: 473–97.

Ahmadi Lewin, F.A. and Thomas, L.E. (2000) "Gerotranscendence and life satisfaction: studies of religious and secular Iranians and Turks," *Journal of Religious Gerontology*, 12: 17–41.

Allen, K.R. and Walker, A.J. (2009) "Theorizing about families and aging from a feminist perspective," in V.L. Bengtson, D. Gans, N.M. Putney, and M. Silverstein (eds) *Handbook of Theories of Aging*, 2nd edn, New York: Springer Publishing Company.

Alvarez, J.T. (1999) *Reflections on an Agequake*, New York: United Nations NGO Committee on Ageing.

Andersen, M.L. and Collins, P.H. (eds) (2007) *Race, Class, & Gender: an Anthology*, 6th edn, Belmont, CA: Wadsworth/Thomson Higher Education.

Arber, S., Davidson, K., and Ginn, J. (2003) "Changing approaches to gender and later life," in S. Arber, K. Davidson, and J. Ginn (eds) *Gender and Ageing: Changing Roles and Relationships*, Maidenhead, U.K.: Open University Press.

Arvidsson, A. (1998) *Livet Som Berattelse. Studier Levnadshistoriska intervjuer*, Lund: Studentlitteratur.

Arvidsson, B. (September 6, 2011) Interview with P. Kolb, Eskilstuna, Sweden.

Atchley, R.C. (1975) "The life course, age grading, and age-linked demands for decision making," in N. Datan and L.H. Ginsberg (eds) *Life-Span Developmental Psychology: Normative Life Crises*, New York: Academic Press.

—— (1993) "Critical perspectives on retirement," in T.R. Cole, W.A. Achenbaum, P.L. Jakobi and R. Kastenbaum (eds) *Voices and Visions of Aging: Toward a Critical Gerontology*, New York: Springer Publishing Company.

—— (1999) *Continuity and Adaptation in Aging: Creating Positive Experiences*, Baltimore, MD: Johns Hopkins University Press.

—— and Barusch, A.S. (2004) *Social Forces and Aging: Creating Positive Experiences*, Belmont, CA: Wadsworth.

Baca Zinn, M., Hondagneu-Sotelo, P., and Messner, M. (2007) "Sex and gender through the prism of difference," in M.L. Andersen and P.H. Collins (eds) *Race, Class, & Gender: An Anthology*, 6th edn, Belmont, CA: Wadsworth/ Thomson Higher Education.

Barthes, R. (1966) *Critique et Verite*, Paris: Editions du Seuil.

Beck, U. (1992) *Risk Society: Towards a New Modernity*, London: Sage.

Bell, D. (1987) *And We Are Not Saved*, New York: Basic Books.

Bengtson, V.L. and Allen, K.R. (1993) "The lifecourse perspective applied to families over time," in P. Boss, W. Doherty, R. LaRossa, W. Schumm and S. Steinmets (eds) *Sourcebook of Family Theories and Methods: A Contextual Approach*, Boston: Allyn and Bacon.

—— Burgess, E.O. and Parrott, T.M. (1997) "Theory, explanation, and a third generation of theoretical development in social gerontology," *Journals of Gerontology: Psychological Sciences and Social Sciences*, 52B: S72–8.

—— Gans, D., Putney, N.M. and Silverstein, M. (2009) "Theories about age and ageing," in V.L. Bengtson, D.Gans, N.M. Putney and M. Silverstein (eds) *Handbook of Theories of Aging*, 2nd edn, New York: Springer Publishing Company.

—— Parrott, T.M. and Burgess, E.O. (1996) "Progress and pitfalls in gerontological theorizing," *Gerontologist*, 36: 768–72.

—— Putney, N.M. and Johnson, M.L. (2005) "The problem of theory in gerontology today," in M.L. Johnson (ed.) *The Cambridge Handbook of Age and Ageing*, Cambridge, U.K.: Cambridge University Press.

—— and Schaie, K.W. (1999) *Handbook of Theories of Aging*, 2nd edn, New York: Springer Publishing Company.

Bernard, J. (1972) *The Future of Marriage*, New York: Bantam.

Biegel, D.E. and Blum, A. (eds) (1990) *Aging and Caregiving: Theory, Research, and Policy*, Newbury Park, CA: Sage.

Birren, J. (1999) "Theories of aging: a personal perspective," in V. Bengtson and K.W. Schaie (eds) *Handbook of Theories of Aging*, 2nd edn, New York: Springer Publishing Company.

—— and Bengtson, V.L. (eds) (1988) *Emergent Theories of Aging*, New York: Springer Publishing Company.

Black, H.K. (2001) "Entering the Storehouse of the Snow: Elders' Narratives of Suffering," unpublished Dissertation, Temple University.

—— (2003) "Narratives of forgiveness in old age," in J.F. Gubrium and J.A. Holstein (eds) *Ways of Aging*, Malden, MA: Blackwell Publishers Ltd.

—— and Rubenstein, R.L. (2000) *Old Souls: Aged Women, Poverty, and the Experience of God*, New York: Aldine deGruyter.

Blytheway, B. (1995) *Ageism*, Buckingham, UK: Open University Press.

Boscoe, A. and Chassard, Y. (1999) "A shift in the paradigm: surveying the European Union discourse on welfare and work," in M. Heikkila (ed.) *Linking Welfare and Work*, Dublin: European Foundation.

Brown, W. (1995) *States of Injury: Power and Freedom in Late Modernity*, Princeton, NJ: Princeton University Press.

Bruner, J. (1986) *Actual Minds, Possible Worlds*, Cambridge, MA: Harvard University Press.

Busse, E. and Maddox, G. (1985) *The Duke Longitudinal Studies of Normal Aging, 1955–1980: Overview of History, Design, and Findings.* NY: Springer Publishing Company.

Butler, J. (1992) "Contingent foundations: feminism and the question of 'postmodernism,'" in J. Butler and J. Scott (eds) *Feminists Theorize the Political*, New York and London: Routledge.

Buckley, W. (1967) *Sociology and Modern Systems Theory*, Englewood Cliffs, NJ: Prentice-Hall.

Calasanti, T. (1996) "Incorporating diversity: meanings, levels of research, and implications for theory," *The Gerontologist*, 36: 147–56.

—— (2003) "Masculinities and care work in old age," in S. Arber, K. Davidson, and J. Ginn (eds) *Gender and Ageing: Changing Roles and Relationships*, Maidenhead, U.K.: Open University Press.

—— (2004) "Feminist gerontology and old men," *Journal of Gerontology* 59B: 305–14.

—— (2009) "Theorizing feminist gerontology, sexuality, and beyond: an intersectional approach," in V.L. Bengtson, D. Gans, N.M. Putney, and M. Silverstein (eds) *Handbook of Theories of Aging*, 2nd edn, New York: Springer Publishing Company.

Calasanti, T. and King, N. (2005) "Firming the floppy penis: age, class, and gender relations in the lives of old men," *Men and Masculinities* 8: 3–23.

Calasanti, T.M. and Slevin, K.F. (2001) *Gender, Social Inequalities, and Aging*, Walnut Creek, CA: Altamira Press.

Calasanti, T. and Zajicek, A. (1993) "A socialist-feminist approach to aging: embracing diversity," *Journal of Aging Studies*, 7: 117–31.

Calhoun, C. (1992) "Changing one's heart," *Ethics*, 103: 76–96.

Cappeliez, P., Beaupre, M., and Robitaille, A. (2008) "Characteristics and impact of life turning points for older adults," *Ageing International*, 32: 54–64.

Coates, J. (2003) *Men Talk: Stories in the Making of Masculinities*, Oxford: Blackwell.

Cohen, J. (1985) "Strategy or identity: new theoretical paradigms in contemporary social movements," *Social Research*, 52: 663–716.

Collins, P.H. (1990) *Black Feminist Thought: Knowledge, Consciousness, and the Politics of Empowerment*, Boston: Unwin Hyman.

Connell, R.W. (1987) *Gender and Power*, Cambridge: Polity Press.

—— (1995) *Masculinities*, Cambridge: Polity Press.

—— (2000) *The Men and the Boys*, Berkeley: University of California Press.

Coombs, W.T. and Holladay, S.J. (1995) "The emerging political power of the elderly," in J.F. Nussbaum and J. Coupland (eds) *Handbook of Communication and Aging*, Hove, UK: Lawrence Erlbaum.

Cumming, E. and Henry, W. E. (1961) *Growing Old: The Process of Disengagement*, New York: Basic Books.

Cumming, E. (1963) "Further thoughts on the theory of disengagement," *UNESCO International Science Journal*, 15: 377–93.

Daatland, S.O. (1997) "Welfare policies for older people in transition? Emerging trends and comparative perspectives," *Scandinavian Journal of Social Welfare*, 6: 153–61.

Dannefer, D. and Kelley-Moore, J.A. (2009) "Theorizing the life course: new twists in the paths," in V.L. Bengtson, D. Gans, N.M. Putney and M. Silverstein (eds) *Handbook of Theories of Aging*, 2nd edn, New York: Springer Publishing Company.

Davey, A., Femia, E.E., Zarit, S.H., Shea, D.G., Sundstroem, G., Berg, S., Smyer, M.A. and Savla, J. (2005) "Life on the edge: patterns of formal and informal help to older adults in the United States and Sweden," *Journal of Gerontology: Psychological Sciences and Social Sciences*, 60B: S281–8.

de Beauvoir, S. (1970) *The Coming of Age*, Paris: Editions Gallimard.

de Beauvoir, S. (1972) *The Second Sex*, Paris: Editions Gallimard.

Delgado, R. (1989) "Storytelling for oppositionists and others: a plea for narrative," *Michigan Law Review*, 87: 2411.

Dilworth-Anderson, P. and Cohen, M.D. (2009) "Theorizing across cultures," in V.L. Bengtson, D. Gans, N.M. Putney and M. Silverstein (eds) *Handbook of Theories of Aging*, 2nd edn, New York: Springer Publishing Company.

Dowd, J. (1975) "Aging as exchange: a preface to theory," *Journals of Gerontology*, 30: 584–94.

Drachman, D. (1992) "A stage-of-migration framework for service to immigrant populations," *Social Work*, 37: 68–72.

Drury, E. (ed.) (1993) *Age Discrimination Against Older Workers in the European Community*, London: Eurolink Age.

—— (ed.) (1997) *Public Policies to Assess Older Workers*, Brussels: Eurolink Age.

Easterlin, R., Schaeffer, C. and Macunovich, D. (1993) "Will the baby boomers be less well off than their parents? Income, wealth, and family circumstances over the life cycle in the United States," *Population and Development Review*, 19: 497–522.

Elder, G.H., Jr. (1974) *Children of the Great Depression*, Chicago: University of Chicago Press.

—— (1999). *Children of the Great Depression*, Boulder, CO: Westview Press.

Erikson, E.H. (1963) *Childhood and Society*, 2nd edn, New York: W.W. Norton & Company.

Erikson, J.M. (1997) *The life cycle completed*, New York: W.W. Norton & Company.

Esping-Andersen, G. (1990) *The Three Worlds of Welfare Capitalism*, Princeton, NJ: Princeton University Press.

—— (1999) *Social Foundations of Postindustrial Economies*, Oxford: Oxford University Press.

Estes, C. (1979) *The Aging Enterprise*, San Francisco: Jossey-Bass Publishers.

—— (1984) *Political Economy, Health, and Aging*, Boston: Little, Brown.

—— (1989) "Aging, health, and social policy: crisis and crossroads," *Journal of Aging and Social Policy*, 1: 17–32.

—— (1991) "The new political economy of aging: introduction and critique," in M. Minkler and C.L. Estes (eds) *Critical Perspectives on Aging: The Political and Moral Economy of Growing Old*, Farmingdale, NY: Baywood.

—— (2006) "Critical feminist perspectives, aging, and social policy," in J. Baars, D. Dannefer, C. Phillipson and A. Walker (eds) *Aging, Globalization, Inequality: The New Critical Gerontology*, Amityville, NY: Baywood Publishing Company, Inc.

—— and Binney, E. (1991) The biomedicalization of aging: dangers and dilemmas, in M. Minkler and C.L. Estes (eds) *Critical Perspectives on Aging: The Political Economy of Growing Old*, Farmingdale, NY: Baywood.

Ewick, P. and Silbey, S.S. (1995) "Subversive stories and hegemonic tales: toward a sociology of narrative," *Law and Society Review*, 29: 197–226.

Fahey, C.J. and Holstein, M. (1993) "Toward a philosophy of the third age," in T.R. Cole, W.A. Achenbaum, P.L. Jakobi and R. Kastenbaum (eds) *Voices and Visions of Aging: Toward a Critical Gerontology*, New York: Springer Publishing Company.

Falconer, W.A. (1923) *Cicero: Se Senectute, De Amicitia, De Divinatione*, Cambridge, MA: Harvard University Press.

Ferraro, K.F., Shippee, T.P. and Schafer, M.H. (2009) "Cumulative inequality theory for research on aging and the life course," in V.L. Bengtson, D. Gans, N.M. Putney and M. Silverstein (eds) *Handbook of Theories of Aging*, 2nd edn, New York: Springer Publishing Company.

Ferree, M.M. and Hall, E.J. (1996) "Rethinking stratification from a feminist perspective: gender, race, and class in mainstream textbooks," *American Sociological Review*, 61: 929–50.

Fischer, R.S., Norberg, A., Lundman, B. (2007) "I'm on my way: the meaning of being oldest old, as narrated by people aged 95 and over," *Journal of Religion, Spirituality & Aging*, 19: 3–19.

Foucault, M. (1977) *Discipline and punish: the birth of the prison*, New York: Vintage.

—— (1978) *The History of Sexuality*, New York: Vintage.

—— (1982) "The subject and power," in H.L. Dreyfus and P. Rabinow (eds) *Michel Foucault: Beyond Structuralism and Hermeneutics*, Chicago: University of Chicago Press.

Frankl, V. (1990) "Facing the transitoriness of human existence," *Generations*, (Fall): 7–10.

Frisby, C. (2004) "Does race matter? Effects of idealized images on African American women's perceptions of body esteem," *Journal of Black Studies*, 34: 323–47.

Garcia-Quinteros, R. (September 5, 2011) Interview with P. Kolb, Eskilstuna, Sweden.

Gergen, M.M. and Gergen, K.J. (2000) "Narratives of the gendered body in popular autobiography," in J.F. Gubrium and J.A. Holstein (eds) *Aging and Everyday Life*, Malden, MA: Blackwell Publishers Ltd.

Giddens, A. (1994) *Beyond Left and Right*, Cambridge, UK: Polity Press.

Gilliland, N. and Havir, L. (1990), "Public opinion and long-term care policy," in D.E. Biegel and A. Blum (eds), *Aging and Caregiving: Theory, Research, and Policy*, Newbury Park, CA: Sage.

Glenngård, A.H., Hjalte, F., Svensson, M., Anell, A. and Bankauskaite, V. (2005) *Health Systems in Transition: Sweden*, Copenhagen: WHO Regional Office for Europe, on behalf of the European Observatory on Health Systems and Policies.

Graham, H. (1984) "Surveying through stories," in C. Bell and H. Roberts (eds) *Social Researching: Politics, Problems, Practice*, London: Routledge & Kegan Paul.

Granberg, E. (September 6, 2011) Interview with P. Kolb, Eskilstuna, Sweden.

Greenberg, S. (2009) *A Profile of Older Americans: 2009*, Washington, D.C.: Administration on Aging, U.S. Department of Health and Human Services.

Gruenberg, E. and Zusman, J. (1964) "The natural history of schizophrenia," *International Psychiatry Clinics* 1: 367–76.

Gubrium, J.F. (1993) "Voice and context in a new gerontology," in T.R. Cole, W.A. Achenbaum, P.L. Jakobi and R. Kastenbaum (eds) *Voices and Visions of Gerontology: Toward a Critical Gerontology*, New York: Springer Publishing Company.

—— (2001) "Narrative, experience, and aging," in G. Kenyon, P. Clark and B. deVries (eds) *Narrative Gerontology: Theory, Research, and Practice*, New York: Springer Publishing Company.

—— (2003) "What Is a Good Story?" *Generations*, 27: 21–4.

—— and Holstein, J.A. (1999) "Constructionist perspectives on aging," in V.L. Bengtson and K.W. Schaie (eds) *Handbook of Theories of Aging*, New York: Springer Publishing Company.

—— and Holstein, J.A. (2000) "Introduction," in J.F. Gubrium and J.A. Holstein (eds) *Aging and Everyday Life*, Malden, MA: Blackwell Publishers, Ltd.

—— and Holstein, J.A. (2003) "Beyond stereotypes," in J.F. Gubrium and J.A. Holstein (eds) *Ways of Aging*, Malden, MA: Blackwell Publishers, Ltd.

—— and Wallace, J. (1990) "Who theorizes age?" in *Aging and Society*, 10: 131–49.

Gutman, D. (1976) "Alternatives to disengagement: the old men of the Highland Druze," in J. Gubrium (ed) *Time, Roles, and Self in Old Age*, New York: Human Sciences Press.

Hagestad, G.O. and Dannefer, D. (2001) "Concepts and theories of aging: beyond microfication in social science approaches," in R.H. Binstock and L.K. George (eds) *Handbook of Aging and the Social* Sciences, 5th edn, San Diego, CA: Academic Press.

Hareven, T. (ed.) (1978) *Transitions: The Family and the Life Course in Historical Perspective*, New York: Academic Press.

—— (1996) (ed.) *Aging and Generation Relations Over the Life Course: A Historical and Cross-Cultural Perspective*, New York: Walter de Gruyter.

—— (2000) *Families, History, and Social Change*. Boulder, CO: Westview.

Havighurst, R.J. (1963) "Successful aging," in R.H. Williams, C. Tibbitts and W. Donahue (eds) *Processes of Aging: Social and Psychological Perspectives*, New York: Atherton.

Heaphy, B., Yip, A.K.T. and Thompson, D. (2004) "Ageing in a non-heterosexual context," *Ageing & Society*, 24: 881–902.

Hendricks, J. (1992) "Generations and the generation of theory in social gerontology," *International Journal of Ageing and Human Development*, 35: 31–47.

Hochschild, A.R. (1976) "Disengagement theory: a logical, empirical, and phenomenological critique," in J.F. Gubrium (ed) *Time, Roles, and Self in Old Age*, New York: Human Sciences Press.

Holtzman, A. (1963) *The Townsend Movement: A Political Study*, New York: Octagon.

Hooyman, N.R. and Kiyak, H.A. (2011) *Social Gerontology: A Multidisciplinary Perspective*, 9th edn, Boston: Allyn & Bacon.

Hutchison, E.D. (2011) "A life course perspective," in E.D. Hutchison (ed) *Dimensions of Human Behavior: The Changing Life Course*, 4rd edn, Los Angeles: Sage Publications.

Hyse, K. and Tornstam, L. (2009) "Recognizing Aspects of Oneself in the Theory of Gerotranscendence," Uppsala: The Social Gerontology Group, Uppsala University. Online. Available HTTP: http://www-old.soc.uu.se/research/gerontology/ (accessed 25 August 2011).

Irving, A. (1999) "Waiting for Foucault: social work and the multitudinous truth(s) of life," in A.S. Chambon, A. Irving and L. Epstein (eds) *Reading Foucault for Social Work*, New York: Columbia University Press.

Jecker, N.S. (1993) "Justice and mother love: toward a critical theory of justice between old and young," in T.R. Cole, W.A. Achenbaum, P.L. Jakobi and R. Kastenbaum (eds) *Voices and Visions of Aging: Toward a Critical Gerontology*, New York: Springer Publishing Company.

Johnson, C.L. and Barer, B.M. (1997) *Life Beyond 85 Years: The Aura of Survivorship*, New York: Springer Publishing Company.

Johnson, M.L. (2005) *The Cambridge Handbook of Age and Ageing*, Cambridge, U.K.: Cambridge University Press.

Jonson, H. (2005) "Social democratic aging in the People's Home of Sweden," *Journal of Aging Studies*, 19: 291–308.

Jung, C.G. (1930, 1982) Die Lebenswende. *Gesammelte Werke 8*, Olten, Germany: Walter-Verlag.

Jung, C.G. (1953) *Collected Works of C.G. Jung, vol. 7*, New York: Pantheon.

Kalache, A., Barreto, S.M. and Keller, I. (2005) "Global ageing: the demographic revolution in all cultures and societies," in M.L. Johnson (ed) *The Cambridge Handbook of Age and Ageing*, Cambridge, U.K.: Cambridge University Press.

Kant, I. (1789) *Foundations of the Metaphysics of Morals*, (Translation by R.P. Wolff, 1969), New York: Bobbs-Merrill.

Kaye, L.W. and Applegate, J.S. (1994) "Older men and the family caregiving orientation," in E.H. Thompson (ed) *Older Men's Lives*, London: Sage.

Kelly, G.A. (1955) *The Psychology of Personal Constructs*, New York: Norton.

Kenyon, G. (1988) "Basic assumptions in theories of human aging," in J. Birren and V. Bengtson (eds) *Emergent Theories of Aging*, New York: Springer Publishing Company.

—— (1997) *Restorying Our Lives: Personal Growth Through Autobiographical Reflection*, Westport, CT: Praeger.

—— G.M., Ruth, J., and Mader, W. (1999) "Elements of a narrative gerontology," in V.L. Bengtson and K.L. Schaie (eds) *Handbook of Theories of Aging*, New York: Springer Publishing Company.

Kimmel, M.S. and Messner, M.A. (eds) (2004) *Men's Lives*, 6th edn, Boston: Pearson/ Allyn & Bacon.

Kinney, J., Stephens, M.A.P., Franks, M.M. and Norris, V.K. (1995) "Stresses and satisfactions of family caregivers of older stroke patients," *Journal of Applied Gerontology*, 14: 3–22.

Kinsella, K. and He, W. (2009) *An Aging World: 2008*, U.S. Census Bureau, International Population Reports, Series P95/09-1, Washington, D.C.: U.S. Government Printing Office.

Kolb, P.J. (2003) *Caring for Our Elders: Multicultural Experiences with Nursing Home Placement*, New York: Columbia University Press.

—— (2008) "Developmental theories of aging," in S.G. Austrian (ed.) *Developmental Theories Through the Life Cycle*, 2nd edn, New York: Columbia University Press.

Kuhn, M. (1972) *Get Out There and Do Something About Injustice*, New York: Friendship Press.

—— (1987) "Politics and aging: the Gray Panthers," in L.L. Carstensen and B.A. Edelstein (eds) *Handbook of Clinical Gerontology*, New York: Pergamon Press.

——, with Long, C. and Quinn, L. (1991) *No Stone Unturned: The Life and Times of Maggie Kuhn*, New York: Ballantine Books.

Kuhn, T.S. (1962) *The Structure of Scientific Revolutions*, New York: Norton.

Kuypers, J.A. and Bengtson, V.E. (1973) "Social breakdown and competence: a model of normal aging," *Human Development*, 16: 181–201.

Landmann, M. (1977) "Foreward," in Z. Tar *The Frankfurt School: The Critical Theories of Max Horkheimer and Theodor W. Adorno*, New York: John Wiley & Sons, Inc.

Levinson, D.J. (1990) "A theory of life structure development in later adulthood," in C.N. Alexander and E.J. Langer (eds) *Higher Stages of Human Development: Perspectives on Adult Growth*, New York: Oxford University Press.

Lilekvist, D. (September 7, 2011) Interview with P. Kolb, Eskilstuna, Sweden.

Lindseth, A. and Norberg, A. (2004) "A phenomenological hermeneutical method for researching lived experience," *Scandinavian Journal of Caring Sciences*, 18: 145–53.

Longino, C.F. and Powell, J.L. (2009) "Toward a phenomenology of aging," in V.L. Bengtson, D. Gans, N.M. Putney and M. Silverstein (eds), *Handbook of Theories of Aging*, New York: Springer Publishing Company.

Luborsky, M.R. and Sankar, A. (1993) "Extending the critical gerontology perspective: cultural dimensions," *The Gerontologist*, 33: 440–4.

Lynott, R.J. and Lynott, P.P. (1996) "Tracing the course of theoretical development in the sociology of aging," *The Gerontologist*, 36: 749–60.

McEwan, E. (ed.) (1990) *Age: The Unrecognised Discrimination*, London: ACE Books.

Mand, K. (2006) "Gender, ethnicity and social relations in the narratives of elderly Sikh men and women," *Ethnic and Racial Studies*, 29: 1057–71.

Mandel, H. and Shalev, M. (2009) "How welfare states shape the gender pay gap: a theoretical and comparative analysis," *Social Forces*, 87: 1873–912.

Mannheim, K. (1952[1928]) "The problem of generations," in P. Kecskmeri (ed.) *Essays in Sociology of Knowledge*, London: Routledge and Kegan Paul.

Marshall, V.W. (1999) "Analyzing social theories of aging," in V.L. Bengtson and K.W. Schaie (eds) *Handbook of Theories of Aging*, 2nd edn, New York: Springer Publishing Company.

—— and Tindale, J.A. (1978) "Notes for a radical gerontology," *International Journal of Ageing and Human Development*, 9: 163–75.

Martin, P., Poon, L.W., Kim, E. and Johnson, M.A. (1996) "Social and psychological resources in the oldest-old," *Experimental Aging Research*, 22: 121–39.

Masui, Y., Gondo, Y., Kawaai, C., Kureta, Y., Takayama, M., Nakagawa, T., Takahashi, R. and Imuta, H. (2010) "The characteristics of gerotranscendence in frail oldest-old individuals who maintain a high level of psychological well-being: a preliminary study using the new gerotranscendence questionnaire for Japanese elderly," *Japanese Journal of Gerontology*, 32: 33–47.

Matsuda, M. (1987) "Looking to the bottom: critical legal studies and reparations," *Harvard Civil Rights-Civil Liberties Law Review*, 22: 323–99.

May, T. and Powell, J. (2008) *Situating Social Theory*, Milton Keynes, UK: McGrawHill.

—— and Williams, M. (2002) *Knowing the Social World*, Milton Keynes, UK: Open University Press.

Meadows, R. and Davidson, K. (2006) "Maintaining manliness in later life: hegemonic masculinities and emphasized femininities" in T. M. Calasanti and K.F. Slevin (eds) *Age Matters: Realigning Feminist Thinking*, New York: Routledge.

Meltzer, B. (2009) "One on one with Dr. Fernando Torres-Gil," THE LINK, the newsletter of the Los Angeles County Commission on Aging, Los Angeles: Los Angeles County Commission on Aging.

Mills, C.W. (1959) *The Sociological Imagination*, New York: Oxford University Press.

Mishler, E.G. (1986) *Research Interviewing: Context and Narrative*, Cambridge, MA: Harvard University Press.

Moody, H. (1988) "Toward a critical gerontology: the contribution of the humanities to theories of aging," in J. Birren and V. Bengtson (eds) *Emergent Theories of Aging*, 2nd edn, New York: Springer Publishing Company.

—— (1993) "Overview: what is critical gerontology and why is it important?" in T.R. Cole, W.A. Achenbaum, P.L. Jakobi and R. Kastenbaum (eds) *Voices and Visions of Aging: Toward a Critical Gerontology*, New York: Springer Publishing Company.

Nakagawa, T., Masui, Y., Kureta, Y., Takayama, M., Takahashi, R. and Gondo, Y. (2011) "The meaning of life in narratives of the oldest old," *Japanese Journal of Gerontology*, 32: 422–33.

Neugarten, B.L. (1964) *Personality in Middle and Late Life: Empirical Studies*, New York: Atherton.

—— (1970) "Dynamics of transition of middle age to old age," *Journal of Geriatric Psychiatry*, 4: 71–87.

—— (1987) "Kansas City Studies of Adult Life," in G.K. Maddox (ed.) *The Encyclopedia of Aging*, New York: Springer Publishing Company.

—— Moore, J.W. and Lowe, J.C. (1965) "Age norms, age constraints, and adult socialization," *American Journal of Sociology*, 70: 710–17.

Nobles, W. (2010) "Understanding the Presence of Gerotranscendence Among Diverse Racial and Ethnic Older Adults in Florida," unpublished dissertation, University of Florida.

Öberg, P. (1997) *Livet Som Berättelse: Om Biografi och Aldrande*, Uppsala: Acta Universitatis Upsaliensis.

Ofstad, H. (1972) *Vart Forakt for Sfaghet: Nazismens Normer Och Varderingar – Och Vara Egna*, Stockholm: Prisma.

Orloff, A.S. (1993) "Gender and the social rights of citizenship: the comparative analysis of gender relations and welfare states," *American Sociological Review* 58: 303–29.

Osgood, N. and McIntosh, J.L. (1986) *Suicide and the elderly*, New York: Greenwood.

Ovrebo, B. and Minkler, M. (1993) "The lives of older women: perspectives from political economy and the humanities," in T.R. Cole, W.A. Achenbaum, P.L. Jakobi and R. Kastenbaum (eds) *Voices and Visions of Aging: Toward a Critical Gerontology*, New York: Springer Publishing Company.

Parsons, T. (1942) "Age and sex in the social structure of the United States," *American Sociological Review*, 7: 604–16.

Pearlin, L.I. (1991) "Life strains and psychological distress among adults," in A. Monat and R.S. Lazarus (eds) *Stress and Coping: An Anthology*, 3rd edn, New York: Columbia University Press.

Peju, M. (September 5, 2011) Interview with P. Kolb, Eskilstuna, Sweden.

Pevik Fasth, J. (September 9, 2011) Interview with P. Kolb, Uppsala, Sweden.

—— and Brandt, T. (2007) "Abstract for *Gerotranscendens I forebyggande halsosamtal*" ["Gerotranscendence in preventive healthcare interviews"], Uppsala: The Social Gerontology Group, Uppsala University. Online. Available http://www.soc.uu.se/en/research/research-fields/the-social-gerontology-group/research/the-theory-of-gerotranscendence/ (accessed 25 August 2011).

Phillipson, C. (2003) "Globalization and the reconstruction of old age: New challenges for critical gerontology," in S. Biggs, A. Lowenstein and J. Hendricks (eds) *The Need for Theory: Critical Approaches to Social Gerontology*, Amityville, NY: Baywood Publishing Company.

Polkinghorne, D. (1988) *Narrative, Knowing and the Human Sciences*, Albany, NY: SUNY Press.

Poon, L.W., Jang, Y., Reynolds, S.G. and McCarthy, E. (2005) "Profiles of the oldest old," in M.L. Johnson (ed.) *The Cambridge Handbook of Age and Ageing*, Cambridge, UK: Cambridge University Press.

—— Sweaney, A.L., Clayton, G.M., Merriam, S.B., Martin, P., Pless, B.S., Johnson, M.A., Thielman, S.B. and Courtenay, B.C. (1992) "The Georgia Centenarian Study," *International Journal of Aging and Human Development*, 34: 1–17.

Prado, C.G. (1995) *Starting with Foucault: An Introduction to Genealogy*, Boulder, CO: Westview Press.

Pratt, H.J. (1976) *The Gray Lobby*, Chicago: University of Chicago Press.

—— (1993) *Gray Agendas: Interest Groups and Public Pensions in Canada, Britain, and the United States*, Ann Arbor, MI: University of Michigan Press.

Putney, N., Alley, D.E. and Bengtson, V.L. (2005) "Social gerontology as public sociology in action," *The American Sociologist*, 36: 88–104.

Quadagno, J. and Street, D. (2006) "Recent trends in U.S. social welfare policy: minor retrenchment or major transformation?" *Research on Aging*, 28: 303–16.

Radina, M.E., Hennon, C.B. and Gibbons, H.M. (2008) "Divorce and mid- and later life families: a phenomenological analysis with implications for family life educators," *Journal of Divorce and Remarriage*, 49: 142–70.

Randall, W. (1995) *The Stories We Are: An Essay on Self-Creation*, Toronto: University of Toronto Press.

Rasmussen, B.H., Sandman, P.O. and Norberg, A. (1995) "Stories about becoming a hospice nurse: reasons, expectations, hopes and concerns," *Cancer Nursing*, 18: 344–54.

Razin, A. and Sadka, E. (2005) *The Decline of the Welfare State: Demography and Globalization*, Cambridge, MA: MIT Press.

Regeringskansliet (Government Offices of Sweden) (2010) "Care of the elderly in Sweden," Online. Available http://www.regeringen.se/sb/d/12073/a/129494 (accessed 15 November 2011).

Renold, E. (2004) "'Other' boys: negotiating non-hegemonic masculinities in the primary school," *Gender and Education*, 16: 247–66.

Riegel, K.F. (1976) "The dialectics of personal development," *American Psychologist*, 31: 689–700.

Riley, M. W. (1986) "The dynamisms of life stages: roles, people, and age," *Human Development*, 29: 150–6.

—— (1987) "On the significance of age in sociology," *American Sociological Review*, 52: 1–14.

—— (1988) (ed) *Social change and the life course*. Beverly Hills, CA.: Sage.

—— (1994) "Aging and society: past, present, and future," *The Gerontologist*, 34: 436–46.

—— Johnson, M. and Foner, A. (1972) *Aging and Society, Vol.3. A Sociology of Age Stratification*, New York: Russell Sage.

—— Kahn, R. and Foner, A. (eds) (1994) *Age and Structural Lag: Society's Failure to Provide Meaningful Opportunities in Work, Family, and Leisure*, New York: Wiley.

—— and Loscocco, K.A. (1994) "The changing structure of work opportunities: towards an age-integrated society," in R.P. Abeles, H.C. Gift and M.G. Ory (eds) *Aging and Quality of Life*, New York: Springer Publishing Company.

—— and Riley, J.W. (1986) "Longevity and social structure: the added years," *Daedalus*, 115: 51–75.

—— and Riley, J.W. (1994) "Structural lag: past and future," in M.W. Riley, R. Kahn and A. Foner (eds) *Age and Structural Lag: Society's Failure to Provide Meaningful Opportunities in Work, Family, and Leisure*, New York: Wiley.

—— and Riley, J.W. (2004) "Age integration and the lives of older people," *The Gerontologist*, 34: 110–15.

Rollins, J. (1995) *All Is Never Said: The Narrative of Odette Harper Hines*, Philadelphia: Temple University Press.

Rosenfeld, D. (2003) "Identity careers of older gay men and lesbians," in J.F. Gubrium and J.A. Holstein (eds) *Ways of Aging*, Malden, MA: Blackwell Publishers Ltd.

Rosow, I. (1976) "Status and role change through the lifespan," in R. Binstock and E. Shanas (eds) *Handbook of Aging and the Social Sciences*, New York: Van Nostrand Reinhold.

Rowe, J. and Kahn, R. (1998) *Successful Aging*. NY: Pantheon.

Rutter, M. (1996) "Transitions and turning points in developmental psychopathology: as applied to the age span between childhood and mid-adulthood," *International Journal of Behavioral Development*, 19: 603–36.

Sanjek, R. (2009) *Gray Panthers*, Philadelphia: University of Pennsylvania Press.

Sadler, E.A., Braam, A.W., Broese van Groenou, M.I., Deeg, D.J.H., and van der Geest, S. (2006) "Cosmic transcendence, loneliness, and exchange of emotional support with adult children: a study among older parents in The Netherlands," *European Journal of Ageing*, 3: 146–54.

Sassen, S. (1991) *The Global City: New York, London, Tokyo*, Princeton, NJ: Princeton University Press.

Schutz, A. (1945) "Some leading concepts of phenomenology," *Social Research*, 12: 77–97.

—— (1967) *The Phenomenology of the Social World*, Evanston: Northwestern University Press.

Settersten, R.A., Jr. and Dobransky, L.M. (2000) "On the unbearable lightness of theory in gerontology," *Gerontologist*, 40: 367–73.

—— and Trauten, M.E. (2009) "The new terrain of old age: hallmarks, freedoms, and risks," in V.L. Bengtson, D. Gans, N.M. Putney and M. Silverstein (eds) *Handbook of Theories of Aging*, 2nd edn, New York: Springer Publishing Company.

Shaskan, G.W. (2009) "Lived Experience of the Old/Old: A Grounded Theory Study of Six San Francisco Bay Area Residents Age 85 Years and Older," unpublished dissertation, The Sanville Institute, Berkeley, CA.

Shea, D., Davey, A., Femia, E.E., Zarit, S.H., Sundstrom, G., Berg, S. and Smyer, M. (2003) "Exploring assistance in Sweden and the United States," *The Gerontologist*, 43: 712–21.

Sherman, E. (2010) *Contemplative aging: a way of being in later life*, New York: Richard Altschuler and Associates.

Smith, D.E. (1987) *The Everyday World as Problematic: A Feminist Sociology*, Boston: Northeastern University Press.

—— (1999) *Writing the Social: Critique, Theory, and Investigations*, Toronto: University of Toronto Press.

Snowden, D. (2001) *Aging with Grace*, Boston: Beacon Press.

Soderberg, S., Lundman, A. and Norberg, A. (1999) "Struggling for dignity: the meaning of living with fibromyalgia," *Qualitative Health Research*, 9: 575–87.

Somers, M.R. (1992) "Narrativity, narrative identity, and social action: rethinking English working-class formation," *Social Science History*, 6: 591–630.

Sorokin, P.A. (1947) *Society, culture and personality*, New York: Harper and Brothers.

Statistics Sweden (2004) "Population prognosis 2004–2050 from the Statistics Sweden." Online. Available http://www.scb.se

—— (2011) "Local taxes." Online. Available http://www.scb.se/Pages/TableAndChart__ 68066.aspx (accessed 16 November 2011).

Stayton, T. (September 5–7, 2011a), Interviews with P. Kolb, Eskilstuna, Sweden.

—— (2011b) "RE: P. Kolb book" E-mail (2 December 2011).

Stein, A. (2008) Feminism's sexual problem: comment on Andersen, *Gender* 22: 115–19.

Stoller, E. and Gibson, R.C. (eds) (2000) *Worlds of Difference: Inequality in the Aging Experience*, 3rd edn, Thousand Oaks, CA: Pine Forge Press.

—— and Gibson, R. C. (2004) "The diversity of American families," in M.L. Andersen and P.H. Collins (eds) *Race, Class, and Gender: An Anthology*, 5th edn, Belmont, CA.: Wadsworth/Thomson Learning.

Stone, R. and Wiener, J. (2001) *Who Will Care for Us? Addressing the Long-Term Care Workforce Crisis*, Washington, D.C.: Urban Institute and the American Association of Homes and Services for the Aging.

Sundin, K., Jansson, L. and Norberg, A. (2002) "Understanding between care providers and patients with stroke and aphasia: a phenomenological hermeneutic inquiry," *Nursing Inquiry*, 9: 93–103.

Tax Rates CC (2011) "Sweden Tax Rates." Online. Available http://www.taxrates.cc/html/sweden-tax-rates.html> (accessed 2 December 2011).

Thorslund, M. (1991) "The increasing number of very old people will change the Swedish model of the welfare state," *Social Science and Medicine*, 32: 455–64.

—— and Silverstein, M. (2009) "Care for older adults in the welfare state: theories, policies, and realities," in V.L. Bengtson, D. Gans, N.M. Putney and M. Silverstein (eds) *Handbook of Theories of Aging*, 2nd edn, New York: Springer Publishing Company.

Thang, L.L. (2000) "Aging in the East: comparative and historical reflections," in T.R. Cole, R. Kastenbaum and R.E. Ray (eds) *Handbook of Aging and the Humanities*, 2nd edn, New York: Springer Publishing Company.

Thomas, P. (2000) "Puerto Rican paradise," in Stoller, E. and Gibson, R.C. (eds), *Worlds of Difference: Inequality in the Aging Experience*, 3rd edn, Thousand Oaks, CA: Pine Forge Press.

Thompson, E.H. (1994) "Older men as invisible in contemporary society," in E.H. Thompson (ed.) *Older Men's Lives*, London: Sage.

Thorsen, K. (1998) "The paradoxes of gerotranscendence: the theory of gerotranscendence in a cultural-gerontological and post-modernist perspective," *Norwegian Journal of Epidemiology*, 8: 165–76.

Thursby, G.R. (2000) "Aging in Eastern religious traditions," in T.R. Cole, R. Kastenbaum and R.E. Ray (eds) *Handbook of Aging and the Humanities*, 2nd edn, New York: Springer Publishing Company.

Tornstam, L. (1989) "Gero-transcendence: a reformulation of the disengagement theory," *Aging*, 1: 55–63.

—— (1992) "The Quo Vadis of gerontology: on the gerontological research paradigm, *The Gerontologist* 32: 318–26.

—— (1997) "Gerotranscendence: The contemplative dimension of aging," *Journal of Aging Studies*, 11: 143–54.

—— (2005) *Gerotranscendence: A Developmental Theory of Positive Aging*, New York: Springer Publishing Company.

—— (September 8, 2011) Interview with P. Kolb, Uppsala, Sweden.

Torres-Gil, F. (2005) "Ageing and public policy in ethnically diverse societies," in M.L. Johnson (ed.) *The Cambridge Handbook of Age and Ageing*, Cambridge, UK: Cambridge University Press.

—— (2011) "RE: 'Ageing and Public Policy in Ethnically Diverse Societies chapter'" E-mail (28 November 2011).

—— and Moga, K.B. (2001) 'Multiculturalism, social policy and the new aging,' *Journal of Gerontological Social Work*, 36: 13–32.

Turner, J.H. (2003) *The Structure of Sociological Theory*, Belmont, CA: Wadsworth/Thomson Learning.

Uhlenberg, P. (2005) "Demography of aging," in P. Uhlenberg (ed.) *Handbook of Population*, New York: Springer Publishing Company.

United Nations (2001) *World Population Ageing: 1950–2050*, New York: United Nations Department of Economic and Social Affairs/Population Division

—— (2002a) "Ageing and development," in *Building a Society for All Ages*, New York: United Nations Department of Economic and Social Affairs/Population Division.

—— (2002b) "Population ageing: facts and figures," in *Building a Society for All Ages*, New York: United Nations Department of Economic and Social Affairs/Population Division.

—— (2002c) "Political Declaration and Madrid International Plan of Action on Ageing," New York: United Nations.

—— (2003) *World Population Prospects: The 2002 Revision*, New York: United Nations Department of Economic and Social Affairs/Population Division.

—— (2009) *World Population Prospects: The 2008 Revision*, New York, United Nations Department of Economic and Social Affairs/Population Division.

—— (2011) "Follow-up to the Second World Assembly on Ageing: Report of the Secretary General," New York: United Nations.

U.S. Department of Labor. (January 2005) *Employment and Earnings*, Washington, D.C.: U.S. Government Printing Office.

Wadensten, B. (2005) "Introducing older people to the theory of gerotranscendence," *Journal of Advanced Nursing*, 52: 381–8.

—— (2007) "The theory of gerotranscendence as applied to gerontological nursing – part I," *International Journal of Older People Nursing*, 2: 289–94.

—— (2010) "Changes in nursing home residents during an innovation based on the theory of gerotranscendence," *International Journal of Older People Nursing*, 5: 108–15.

—— and Carlsson, M. (2007a) "The theory of gerotranscendence in practice: guidelines for nursing – part II," *International Journal of Older People Nursing*, 2: 295–301

—— and Carlsson, M. (2007b) "Adoption of an innovation based on the theory of gerotranscendence by staff in a nursing home – part III," *International Journal of Older People Nursing*, 2: 302–14.

—— and Hagglund, D. (2006) "Older people's experience of participating in a reminiscence group with a gerotranscendental perspective: reminiscence group with a gerotranscendental perspective in practice," *International Journal of Older People Nursing*, 1: 159–67.

Walker, A. (1990) "The economic 'burden' of aging and the prospect of intergenerational conflict," *Ageing and Society*, 10: 377–96.

—— (1997) *Combating Age Barriers in Employment*, Luxembourg: Office for the Official Publications of the European Communities.

—— (2002, September) *Cultures of ageing – a critique*, Paper presented to the British Society of Gerontology Annual Conference, Birmingham, UK.

—— (2006) "Reexamining the political economy of aging: understanding the structure/agency tension," in J. Baars, D. Dannefer, C. Phillipson and A. Walker (eds) *Aging, Globalization, and Inequality: The New Critical Gerontology*, New York: Baywood Publishing Company.

—— (2009) "Commentary: the emergence and application of active aging in Europe," *Aging and Social Policy*, 21: 75–93.

—— and Guillemard, A.M. and Alber, J. (1993) *Older People in Europe: Social and Economic Policies*, Brussels: Commission of the European Communities.

—— and Naegele, G. (eds) (1999) *The Politics of Old Age in Europe*. Buckingham, U.K.: Open University Press.

Wallace, S.P., and Williamson, J.B. (1992) *The Senior Movement: References and Resources*, New York: G.K. Hall.

Wang, F.T.Y. (1999) "Resistance and old age: the subject behind the American seniors' movement," in A.S. Chanbon, A. Irving and L. Epstein (eds) *Reading Foucault for Social Work*, New York: Columbia University Press.

Werner, C.A. (2011). *The older population: 2010: 2010 census briefs*. U.S. Department of Commerce, Economics and Statistics Administration, U.S. Census Bureau.

White, H. (1987) *The Content of the Form*, Baltimore: Johns Hopkins University Press.

Whitehead, S.M. (2002) *Men and Masculinities: Key Themes and New Directions*, Cambridge, U.K.: Polity Press.

Williamson, J.B., Evans, L. and Powell, L.A. (1982) *The Politics of Aging: Power and Policy*, Springfield, IL: Charles C. Thomas.

Wolf, M. (1975) "Women and suicide in China," in M. Wolf and R. Witke (eds) *Women in Chinese Society*, Palo Alto, CA: Stanford University Press.

World Health Organization (2002) *Active Ageing: A Policy Framework*, Geneva: World Health Organization.

—— (2007) *Global Age-friendly Cities: A Guide*, Geneva: World Health Organization.

—— (2009) "WHO Global Network of Age-Friendly Cities," Geneva: World Health Organization. Online. Available http://www.who.int/ageing/Brochure-EnglishAFC9.pdf (accessed 14 November 2011).

—— (2011) "First International Age-friendly Cities Conference," Geneva: World Health Organization. Online. Available http://www.who.int/ageing/en/ (accessed 14 November 2011).

Young, I.M. (1990) *Justice and the Politics of Difference*, Princeton, NJ: Princeton University Press.

Zusman, I. (1966) "Some explanations of the changing appearance of psychotic patients: antecedents of the social breakdown syndrome concept," *Milbank Memorial Fund Quarterly*, 44: 363–94.

Index

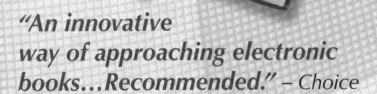
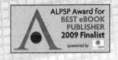
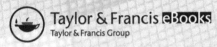

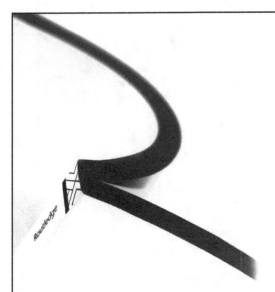
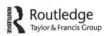

Printed in the United States
by Baker & Taylor Publisher Services

Printed in the United States
by Baker & Taylor Publisher Services